Wombology

Wombology

✦

Healing the Primordial Memories and Wounds Your Grandmother's Daughther Gave To You

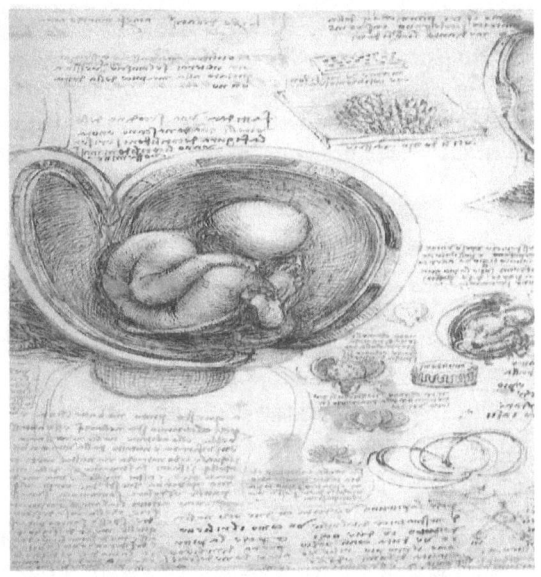

C J Johnson, PsyD

iUniverse, Inc.

New York   Bloomington

Wombology

Healing the Primordial Memories and Wounds Your Grandmother's Daughther Gave To You

iUniverse books may be ordered through booksellers or by contacting:

iUniverse
1663 Liberty Drive
Bloomington, IN 47403
www.iuniverse.com
1-800-Authors (1-800-288-4677)

ISBN: 978-0-595-49692-1 (pbk)
ISBN: 978-0-595-49427-9 (cloth)
ISBN: 978-0-595-61212-3 (ebk)

Printed in the United States of America

iUnivers rev. date: 1/16/2009

This book is dedicated with love, gratitude, and respect to all the mothers who walked this path before me and especially to the members of my seven generations:

- My mother, the Reverend Geraldine B. Jenkins
- My grandmothers, Nellie Burton and Melinda Curry
- My great-grandmothers Annie Noble Peppars and LuCandy Jenkins
- My great-great-grandmother Charity Noble

To my husband, Harold Keith, son, Roddrick, daughter, Chakira, and my sister, Linda Colbert, I appreciate all that you do. And to my late father L C Jenkins.

Contents

Acknowledgments

Heartfelt gratitude and appreciation go to all those who played a part in completing this project:

The Reverend Geraldine Jenkins, my mother, for planting and nurturing the seeds of faith, trust, and love for an eternal God deep within me during my wombology. She is truly an earth angel. Her anointed healing oils of patience, forgiveness, love, support, and empathy are etched deep within my soul. I am blessed and indebted. L C Jenkins, my father (who crossed over in 2004) for planting seeds of strength, integrity, and healthy boundaries.

My immediate family, Harold Keith, Roddrick, and Chakira, for pushing me to finish this project and bring it into the world to help others heal.

Linda Colbert, my sister, for co-facilitating wombology workshops and making sure I stay on target during workshops and the writing of this book. To my brothers, Larry Clyde and Jimmy Ray Jenkins, for being there for me.

Dr. Christiane Northrup, for writing her book *Mother-Daughter Wisdom*, which touched me deeply and contributed to the writing of this book. Dr. Eva Shaw's encouraging words and nudges.

My editorial team: Rachel Derowitsch, Chakira Johnson, Linda Colbert, and Ann Roney.

iUniverse partners: from the editors to the printers, I appreciate all of your efforts.

To past and current clients who are my teachers of the human spirit's resilience. And for those who planted the seed for this book by permitting me to bear witness to their most intimate moments.

List of Figures

A Special Note to the Reader

The material presented in this book is intended to open the discussion for the concept of *wombology, how a pregnant woman's deep, persistent emotional state can significantly affect the development of temperament, personality, and character of her unborn child. This shaping of the unborn's consciousness can last throughout the life span.* The word *wombology* is my personal idiom for which I have been awarded a copyright for the next ninety-five years.

Professionals have differing opinions about the theories presented within this book. The worksheets, treatments, and techniques I include or suggest should be undertaken with the guidance of your healthcare practitioner or psychotherapist, especially if you are already in therapy or considering it. If my truth seems inscrutable, then consider Edward de Bono's investigative PMI attitude, from the book *de Bono's Thinking Course*, which asks these questions: What is the *plus* of this theory? What is the *minus* of this theory? And what is *interesting* about this theory? This attitude will enable you to be open to at least taking into consideration what you are reading, hearing, or experiencing. Ask yourself, what would be the plus in this theory for me? What would be the minus in this theory for me? And what would be most interesting about this wombology theory for me? Maybe this will lead to new information about you; maybe it could explain what has been unexplainable. In addition, ask yourself, What about this alternative view could work for me? An open mind and heart will generate new possibilities and choices. If you can change your mind, you can change yourself.

Acronyms and Their Meanings

SEMP — Spiritual, Emotional, Mental, Physical
FOOLISH —Family Of Origin Lies I Still Hear
VFOS — Vaginal Fallout Syndrome
CYSB — Call Your Spirit Back
FOO — Family of Origin
LSI— Life Scene Investigation
PAST—Put Away Stifling Things
SMART—Specific, Measurable, Achievable, Related to a goal, Time-limited

Introduction

Tears filled my eyes every day for the first two weeks of my psychology internship for the University of Southern Colorado at the Colorado State Hospital. My husband would ask me if I had chosen the right profession since I was always tearful when I got home. I was working with preteens and teens who were living in the locked-up units at the Colorado State Hospital. My tears were for their pain and wounds received from families so dysfunctional they had imploded. This was in 1993. After seventeen years of retail sales and ten years of teaching aerobic exercise, I had started my pursuit of my bachelor of science degree in psychology at age thirty-six in 1990.

In 1994 I graduated with honors and with unexpected insight into why many people choose psychology as a major (to heal their wounds). Back then; I was naïve enough to think everyone was pursuing the degree for altruistic reasons.

In 1995 I was working in Parkview Medical Center's behavioral units; that is where I realized I could not continue to work in the children's unit. The children tugged at my heart too much, and I did not want to continue to be overwhelmed by their wounds while I was pursuing my master of arts in psychology. I decided working and completing my externship in the Chemical Dependency Unit (CDU) would be less taxing emotionally. By the time I graduated from the University of Northern Colorado with my master's degree, I realized CDU was the right choice. Working with addicts is quite challenging but indeed rewarding, especially when they find sobriety.

In May 2000 I had been shelter manager of a battered woman's center for six months when I became the therapist for the center's victims of domestic violence. I also began to pursue a doctorate. In 2003, when I graduated from

Southern California University for Professional Studies with my doctorate in psychology (PsyD), I had developed my wombology theory with one of my adoptee clients. (A disproportionate number of my victims of domestic violence clients were adoptees.) I started paying attention to their stories of coming into the world feeling sad, abandoned, or guilty about something and not knowing why. The feelings of abandonment, guilt, and sadness became the code words for me to ask about wombology. As I compared stories, most of my clients were a result of unwanted pregnancies. This gave me clearer insights as to why they came into the world already harboring emotions they could not explain.

The psychology of healing is my passion and the driving force behind this book. The dynamics between generations of mother and child are most intriguing to me.

Sometimes I use the phrase "grandmother's daughter" instead of "mother." The phrase alone makes a person stop and ask, "Who is that?" It asks the person to look at his or her mother differently. Dr. Christiane Northrup's use of the phrase in her book *Mother-Daughter Wisdom* made me catch my breath and mentally acknowledge that there was a point in my mother's life when she was a daughter. This phrase has had the same effect on my clients and workshop participants. During workshops when I say "grandmother's daughter," most participants laugh at themselves because it takes a minute before it sinks in who we are discussing.

I have been in private practice for five years in the Atlanta, Georgia, area. I offer individual, couples, and group therapy. My favorite type of "couple" to work with is mother-daughter. It is an intriguing dynamic to be a part of and to witness, including my own as a daughter and as a mother to a daughter. Father-son is my next favorite couple; the dynamics within that relationship are so different from mother-daughter but just as intriguing. In therapy sessions, I concentrate on the exploration of spiritual, emotional, mental, and physical aspects of each client to help them find emotional balance and alignment.

This book is based on my clinical observations and on the research I examined in an effort to present more than just my theory. I expect some scientists, physicians, and others to scoff at my theory. I have been met with strong declarations of, "I don't buy that for a minute," to a simple "interesting"—even as their body language offers a different message. I have felt the anger of those whose toes I may be stepping on and who will not accept or receive the possibility of wombology, despite the scientific evidence on record by scientists decades before me.

In this book you will learn about Dr. Lester Sontag and his study on how the Great Depression affected pregnant women and their babies. And you will discuss Dr. Thomas Verny's journey into the life of the unborn through his book written in the 1980s.

Ninety percent of the people I discuss the theory of wombology with receive, explore, understand, and accept the possibility of it as a truth. In this book you will find the stories and experiences that I have encountered, as I have not designed, initiated, or carried out an empirical experiment or study to prove or disprove the theory. I believe it to be very real. Twenty years ago the words *Internet*, *e-mail*, and *World Wide Web* were not household words. Today, they are household and global words. Can you imagine life without them now? I use e-mail every single day to communicate by simply typing a message and then hitting the Send button. I cannot explain and I do not even understand the intricate details of how cyberspace works, but that does not stop me from using it.

Maybe wombology will be like e-mail for many people: something they do not understand completely but know that it does affect daily life. My guess is that 80 percent of the time we do not know what happens during the healing process. How much does the "how" matter? I have found that what works for one person may not work for another. If I can help 80 percent of the people I touch, I am okay with the 20 percent who choose not to heal.

My main purpose in life is to help the weary and wounded who want to stop picking at their emotional scabs and are ready for emotional health and freedom. This often means helping to make the invisible visible, to kick the uninvited guests of shame and guilt out, to give voice to the unexplained, and to stop the circular rational lies of denial that holds onto the unexamined past. And as a spirit-led and spirit-fed (obedient to Divine Spirit's insight and directives) psychologist, I help those who are trying to understand what is out of alignment in life, why the heart and actions are incongruent, and how to establish and maintain harmony.

I've written this book to acknowledge and validate the unnamed and unclaimed pain from the first environment, to help heal those deep wounds received in the womb. Too often primordial wounds and memories become generational curses, pain, and confusion that need to be explored, not continued inadvertently. Many Native American Indians believe that we each are responsible for seven generations. I wholeheartedly agree and accept my responsibility. If one generation can become whole, it is healing for all the others. It is worth the time, energy, and effort it takes to heal.

If after reading this book you find a way to live each day as if it affects your tomorrow, you will be living a purpose-filled life, and the people in your seven generations will be given that same choice too. Clarifying what is yours and what is not yours will open up possibilities for you to soar to the peaks of unimagined personal heights and growth.

To your emotional freedom,

Dr. C J

Your embryonic state is not your final fate

1

Womb-time Can Dictate a Lifetime

✦

Uook, Uook, Uook. I have to walk away from the skillet of eggs I'm trying to scramble before I throw up. Three months ago I could scramble eggs without invoking the gag reflex. But now I'm three months pregnant and going through all the hormonal changes that entails.

That was more than thirty years ago. To this day my husband will ask this question to our son and get the same answer. "Roddy, I'm scrambling some eggs. How many do you want?"

"Dad, I don't really care for scrambled eggs, for the fifteenth zillionth time. Gees, you have known me for thirty-one years and I have never liked scrambled eggs. When will you get it?"

My husband usually responds with, "Oh, I forgot. So sue me!"

I have witnessed this exchange more times than I care to remember, but just this month, I made the connection and now realize that my thirty-three-year-old son communicated to me his dislike of scrambled eggs while he was in my womb by causing the gag reflex every time I looked at eggs being scrambled. After he was born I had no problems with cooking or eating scrambled eggs. What did I crave while pregnant with him? Whataburger cheeseburgers and french fries. Can you imagine what his favorite foods are today? You guessed it, cheeseburgers and fries. Roddy's first complete sentence when he was a toddler was, "This ain't the way to McDonald's."

I listened to Marvin Gaye, the late, great rhythm and blues (R&B) singer-song writer, all the time when I was pregnant with Roddy, my firstborn. I remember him kicking and moving around a lot in the womb when I would dance to or play Marvin's music. I can remember my son's little fat calves dipping up and down and bouncing to the beat when he was a few months old and just beginning to pull himself up on the 1970s chocolate brown, crushed velvet sofa's edge whenever I played Marvin. It was his happy music while in the womb, and today Marvin Gaye remains one of our all-time favorite entertainers.

These incidents are not empirical evidence for my Wombology theory, but anecdotal experiences can put the concept on the conversation table. *Wombology is the belief that a pregnant woman's deep, persistent or constant emotional state can significantly affect the development of temperament, character, and personality traits of her unborn child. This shaping of the unborn child's consciousness can last throughout the life span.* The operative word in this concept is *can*. I am not proposing that every emotion a pregnant woman experiences will permanently affect her unborn child, but I am proposing that when an unborn child is constantly exposed to and experiences certain emotions with the mother, those emotions and/or behaviors can become a part of the infant's implicit memory. My theory situates itself as the true first stage of development. Could it be the missing link or an expanded explanation for all other theories of development? Yes, I think so.

Wombology affects three main aspects of a person: temperament, character, and personality. Temperament is defined as the individual's stable manner of behavior or reaction. Character is defined as the distinctive attributes that make or distinguish an individual. Personality is defined as the expression of the four dimensions of self—spiritual, emotional, mental, and physical—that bring continuity to an individual's behavior in different situations and at different times. Personality changes and is shaped by internal needs and external pressure over time. These definitions are descriptions that I have gleaned, accepted, and paraphrased over time and are operational for me.

Since 2001, when this theory first started percolating in my mind, nine out of ten of my clients, whom I have presented the theory to finds some validity in it, either for their own wombology/life story or in recognizing their child's personality from their pregnancy experience. The theory explains a part of the client's mother that was not understandable or that he or she was unaware of before.

Just this week, while noshing on my favorite part of a fried pork chop—the bone—it hit me: this is what I did while pregnant with Chakira, my last-born. Today, thirty years later, my daughter's favorite meat is pork chops. Chewing on the bone while we sit at the dinner table and talk is one of our rituals. I craved okra while pregnant with her, and her favorite vegetable is okra. I craved ice as well, and Chakira loves to chew on ice. Here again, these examples are not proof but are certainly worth discussing.

I called my mom up three days ago and asked her if she remembers what she craved when she was pregnant with me. She said, " Girl, do you know how long ago that was? Well, the first thing that comes to mind is lemon." I *love* lemons. They have always been my favorite fruit to eat; I like them with salt and peppermint candy. My mouth waters at the thought of it right now. The delicious habit of continually eating lemons when I was a child resulted in a loss of tooth enamel and lots of fillings as an adult. As a matter of fact, Mom would not let me eat lemons while I was pregnant. She said, "You don't know what all that acid could be doing to your baby!" Hmmm. Here we go again.

Research shows that many chemical compounds and products of the mother's diet cross the placenta, providing the fetus with a changing range of tastes and smells. Dr. David B. Chamberlain states, "The structures for tasting are available at about 14 weeks g.a. and experts believe that tasting begins at that time. Tests show that swallowing increases with sweet tastes and decreases with bitter and sour tastes. In the liquid womb space, a range of tastes are presented including lactic, pyruvic, and citric acids… Tests made at birth reveal exquisite taste discrimination and definite preferences."[1] Therefore, if most of what a mother eats, drinks, or consumes is passed through her bloodstream into the body of her baby, it makes sense that if the fetus and mom can share food likes and dislikes, they could share emotional states as well. The maternal emotional states are transferred physiologically, as well as through hormones. I am not the first to propose this intimate connection between mother and baby before birth. But I do believe it is my turn to speak its truth.

Dr. Thomas Verny's quest or inquiry into the life of the unborn started in 1975. In 1981 he and John Kelly wrote *The Secret Life of the Unborn Child*, in which they told of the possibilities that the parents' (both mom and dad) preconception attitudes can affect the development of the unborn child. For example, if a woman wants to become pregnant, her attitude will be totally different when the test comes back positive than if she did not want a baby or feel that she was not ready to be a parent.[2] Twenty-seven years after Dr. Verny's book, I am submitting a continuation of observations of how the life of the unborn child still is important to all concerned.

Dr. Paul Pearsall, author of *The Heart's Code: Tapping the Wisdom and Power of Our Heart Energy*, says, "The fetus' heart also influences the heart of the mother and less so the father. The possibility of 'L' (info-energy of the heart's code) energy radiated from the embryo may help explain the creation of an energetic dialogue and information feedback system that contributes to the creation of not only the temperament of the child but changes in temperament of the mother, the father, and the entire family when a new heart emerges among old hearts."[3] This makes sense to me and explains how a woman can enjoy something before pregnancy, hate it during pregnancy, and then enjoy it again after pregnancy.

It is still widely believed that we humans are a blank slate until we exit the womb, but research now agrees with what most mothers have known intuitively: the unborn has the capacity to perceive and remember sounds of speech, to recognize a story heard repeatedly in utero, to bounce to the beat of music it heard repeatedly, and to recognize its own mother's voice. The unborn baby forms the brain structures necessary for learning and awareness by the twenty-eighth week. Many prenatal psychologists, such as the members of the International Society of Prenatal and Perinatal Psychology and Medicine (ISPPM) of Germany, acknowledge that the core of human personality forms in the womb.[4] During the 16th International Congress on "The Anthropology and Psychology of Pregnancy and Birth in 2005, Austrian psychoanalyst Alfons Reiter stated, "Prenatal attachment and relationship processes predetermine the capacity to relate and methods of bonding in later life."[5]

Humans go through three main stages before we exit the womb, or separate from mom as an infant. First, the zygote is the cell that forms with the union of the sperm and ovum at conception. Second, the embryo is the prenatal organism from two to eight weeks after conception, during which our body structures and internal organs develop. Third, the fetus (unborn child) is the prenatal organism from the beginning of the third month to the end of pregnancy, when infancy begins.

The late Carl Upchurch discussed the negative emotional states he received in the womb in his appropriately titled book, *Convicted in the Womb: One Man's Journey from Prisoner to Peacemaker*. Upchurch realized it was through his unconscious mind, not his DNA, that he received the violent tendencies and negativity in the womb. This knowledge helped him to move beyond his own story of wombology. During one of his ten-year stays within Pennsylvania's "gated community" (penal system), he received this insight. It took him years to make the adjustment and change to being a different type of person. (I know from personal and clinical experiences that too often wisdom comes gift wrapped in pain.)

Nevertheless, Upchurch was able to overcome his wombology. He wrote, "I saw the possibility of extricating myself from feelings of worthlessness and despair, self-denunciation and disrespect, emotional self-loathing and purposeful self-denial."[6] He was able to refocus the programming he received in the womb from the moment his soul entered his body. He channeled his rage-filled energy into helping others and earned a national reputation as a peacemaker between rival gangs across our nation before his untimely death in 2003.

The King James Version of the Bible refers to the womb at least seventy times, and it talks about two nations and two manner of people being in the womb of one woman (Gen. 25:23). It discusses hiding in the inner chamber (1 Kings 22:25), and my favorite is from Jer. 1:5, "Before I formed thee in the belly I knew thee; and before thou camest forth out of the womb I sanctified thee...[7] If back in biblical days (when men and their actions were much more prominent than women) this part of a woman's body was important enough to discuss at least seventy times, I think we need to take another look at this ever-present, life-giving chamber of a woman's body. I will tell you about my grandmother's daughter's affect on me in the womb later.

I worked as a psychotherapist with victims of domestic violence for four years here in Henry County, Georgia. My first conscious insight into what I now call wombology came in 2001 with Stephanie, a domestic violence victim during a therapy session. She kept saying, "C J, I have felt guilty about everything all of my life, and I don't even know why. I feel like I carry enough guilt for the whole world." When she couldn't explain why she had always felt that way I was baffled, until the next session when she told me she was adopted. Ah-ha, it made sense to me now.

I told her, "You have carried your biological mother's emotions that she felt while pregnant with you." In the early 1960s, some forty years ago, there still was stigma attached to a young high school girl getting pregnant out of wedlock, especially in the small town in Michigan where Stephanie was conceived, born, and given up for adoption. That revelation helped me to understand how we can be intimately and eternally connected to our biological mothers and not be aware of the connections.

Fast forward to 2007. A few months ago we found Stephanie's biological mother. As they build their relationship, we have found that the emotional states Stephanie always had and could not explain were confirmed by her bio-mother, Grace. Her bio-mother welcomed Stephanie finding her and wanted her daughter to know that she was given away in the spirit of love and what she thought was the best for both of them. Even though Stephanie and Grace are just now finding each other again, their emotional relationship and Stephanie's emotional self started during her womb-time.

I was at the first meeting between these two women and watched these two spirits hug each other and explore each other's faces and bodies, looking for similarities. This was the first time Grace got to touch her baby she had given birth to some forty years ago. In the home for the unwed mothers where Grace had stayed, staff would not allow the mothers to hold the infant. They were permitted only to look at them through thick-paned glass for fifteen minutes, and that was it. So when we were winding up the meeting,

Grace went through the anxiety of giving up Stephanie all over again. That was one of my most moving moments with a client.

Dr. Christiane Northrup tells us in her mind-blowing book (which inspired this book) *Mother-Daughter Wisdom: Creating a Legacy of Physical and Emotional Health*, "Every woman is a daughter. A woman's health is the soil out of which all humanity grows. Enhancing a woman's health fertilizes and replenishes this soil for everyone—men, women, children, plants, animals, and the planet itself. The mother-daughter bond in all its beauty, pain, and complexity forms the very foundation of a woman's state of health. This primal relationship leaves its mark on every cell of our being throughout our lives."[8] I love that and cannot agree with her more. She also tells us that in the case of an adoption, the minute the mothers are switched the baby knows on some cellular level that her mother has been switched. I support this theory and propose that when the mother decides to give the unborn baby up for adoption, the unborn baby receives that message in the womb. And that may explain why it is so difficult for some adopted children to outgrow the feeling that something is missing or that something is wrong with them. In addition, the feeling of abandonment becomes an emotional staple.

At least 70 percent of my domestic violence clients were adoptees, and most of them struggled with the sense that they were a little crazy. No matter how wonderful their adopted parents were, something just did not feel right; they often did not feel as if they actually belonged to their family.

If you are adopted and feel this way, you are not crazy. It's just that your inner world (first environment) did not continue to match your outer world.

One adoptee client, Jon, said, "I always felt like a one-eyed alien because I did not look like 'my' family. I always felt like an outsider looking in, and I did not know until much later in life that I was adopted." He also told me, "C J, I always thought I was either insane or an alien, and being an alien was easier for me to deal with than being insane." Jon later found his biological mother and wished he had not, because she did not match his dream mom. And with a nervous chuckle he said, "The family tree is full of nuts and would make a great *Jerry Springer* episode. As a matter of fact, it would be great for ratings week."

At one of my husband's family gatherings a couple of years ago, I was watching a young mom give her infant son to his father while she went to visit the ladies' room. While she was gone the baby became restless and cranky. The father could not soothe him, so other female relatives tried to soothe the little one until Mom got back. It worked for a second until the baby rubbed his nose against the woman's chest; then he would cry again. When Mom came back and the baby rubbed his nose against Mom's chest, all was well—no more cranky, fidgety baby. That observation led me to the phrase, "in search of Mama's scent," because the baby knew that all the other women who handled him did not smell like, sound like, or feel like his mom, which increased his discomfort.

So imagine being attuned to one woman's rhythms, voice, and food likes and dislikes carried through the placenta before birth and through the breast milk after birth for those who were breast-fed. For nine months an infant has been as one with her bio-mother, and then after fighting its way through the birth canal, nothing matches what she already knows as a natural part of her. Can you understand the feeling of being a foreigner in your own skin and not knowing why?

That age-old warning given to pregnant women when I was growing up, "Girl, you are going to mark your baby," means a lot more to me now within the context of wombology. According to Dr. Verny and many other researchers, what seems to matter most during pregnancy is how the mother feels about her unborn child.

Right after finishing my undergrad in psychology in 1994, I worked on the children and adolescent unit at a hospital in Pueblo, Colorado. One question on the intake form, the questionnaire used to gather information about a new patient, intrigued me. "Was this child a product of a wanted pregnancy?" At first I couldn't figure out why I had to ask a mother this question. I asked an experienced co-worker about this, and she explained, "Girl, if she didn't want the baby in her stomach, she usually doesn't want the baby after 'it' is born and she will treat the baby as if it is a bother. Most of the children we see have emotional and behavior problems and are from an unwanted pregnancy."

My co-worker was right. I had noticed when I asked this question that many of the mothers would laugh and say, "It wasn't planned, but she's here now … oh, well." So, the disconnect many adoptees feel makes even more sense as I learn more about the mother-child bond in utero and the development of the emotional self while in the womb.

Upchurch wrote, "I spent all of my childhood, and way too much of my adulthood, trying to stimulate a caring response from her" (his mother). Of course, I believe this detached relationship started while Upchurch was in utero. I wonder how many people are going through what I call the FOOLISH (family of origin lies I still hear) ghost dance and disconnection like Upchurch experienced. The FOOLISH ghost dance implies that today you are still reacting to the family lies or untruths in the same way you did as a child and therefore continuing the dysfunctional family or tribal ritual of going nowhere but in a vicious circle.

I had a client whose mother was an in-home prostitute, and this boy was told he was dirty and would never amount to anything but a male slut. He talked about the smells and sounds of his childhood, which still haunt him. I explained some of that was from the womb and that he is still doing the

FOOLISH ghost dance. When I was growing up, some relatives often told me that I would not amount to much either. If I still believed that family of origin lie, I would be stuck in my own emotional muck and would not be doing what I am doing now. Family untruths are usually someone else's projection of unresolved pain. Only wounded people purposely wound others. Most people who have some of those deep wounds do not want to deal with their pain because deep wounds require time, energy, and deep healing. No matter what the pain is, you cannot heal what you cannot feel.

A baby's first environment is the most important environment when it comes to successfully moving through childhood developmental stages into adulthood. Long before they are born, before they can put a meaning on events or understand what is going on, babies are beings who think, feel, and remember. That is why what happens before birth profoundly influences the person that baby will become. In his book *The Secret Life of the Unborn Child*, Dr. Verny wrote, "The fetus can see, hear, experience, taste and, on a primitive level, even learn *in utero* (that is, in the uterus—before birth). Most importantly, he can *feel*—not with an adult's sophistication, but feel nonetheless."[9]

Health Media Ltd. reported that researchers from Queen's University in Canada and Zhejiang University in China published a study in the journal *Psychological Science* (2003) that showed that the fetus is capable of learning in the womb and can remember and recognize his mother's voice. Dr. Barbara Kisilevsky, lead researcher of that study, said, "This is an extremely exciting finding that provides evidence for sustained attention, memory, and learning by the fetus." Kisilevsky also stated that the findings showed that what babies' experience in the womb affected their behavior and development and that voice recognition may play a role in mother-infant attachment.[10]

As part of this study, mothers read poetry to their unborn. When a fetus heard his mother's voice, his heart rate accelerated, while the heart rate of a fetus who heard a stranger's voice would go down significantly. Dr. Anthony DeCasper, developmental researcher at the University of North Carolina, Greensboro, Dr. David B. Chamberlain, founding editor of birthpsychology. com, and many other researchers believe the foundations for speech perception and language acquisition are laid before birth and the beginnings of specific languages from their mothers' start while in the womb.[11] Research using acoustic spectroscopy, a noninvasive device that makes detailed printouts of sound, much like a fingerprint, has shown that a baby's cry already contains some of her mother's speech rhythms and voice characteristics.[12]

Dr. Lester Sontag, the first director for the Fels Longitudinal Study, which started in 1929 to determine the effects of the Great Depression on child development, demonstrated in the 1930s and 1940s that, "Maternal attitudes and feelings could leave a permanent mark on the unborn child's personality."[13] Dr. Sontag also was the first scientist to recognize that the mother's heartbeat affected the heartbeat of the unborn child in the womb in many ways. He called his theory "somatopsychics." Studies have shown that the mother's heart rate is the baby's measuring stick for safety, inside and outside the womb. It takes seconds for the mother's heart rate to register with the unborn and for the unborn to react to it.

The National Geographic Channel broadcast a series of programs in 2005 titled *In the Womb*. In the first one, the three-dimensional and four-dimensional ultrasound imagery was used to follow one woman throughout her nine-month pregnancy. It is mind-boggling what those images were able to let us experience along with the expecting mom and unborn baby. For example, at eleven weeks you can see her sucking her preferred thumb, which prepares her for right- or left-handedness in the outside world. The unborn is in total darkness in the womb, yet you watch the fetus open and close her eyes. At twelve weeks she starts the blinking reflex. And the imagery shows her reacting to her mother's emotional state, physical actions, and food that she ate.[14] I highly recommend this DVD. It would make a great gift for expectant mothers or to add to your resource library. The other programs covered the gestation periods of multiple births and animals.

Dr. Sontag's empirical evidence supported his theory that what was going on in the world affected the mother and her unborn child. His conclusion was that the pervasive fears of the pregnant women heightened children's biological susceptibility to emotional distress while still in the womb. Since that time we have had so many profound national disasters and events that caused pervasive fears that we can pick a year to study and replicate his findings.

The popular names of newborns at any given time period show how the external world affects the internal world of the pregnant woman. For instance, how many men do you know who are in their forties who are named John Fitzgerald? Remember, President John Fitzgerald Kennedy was shot in 1963, and many mothers honored his life by naming their sons after him. How many women do you know in the same age group who are named Jacquelyn in honor of the First Lady? Each generation has its catastrophic event that becomes a flash bulb memory (I'll write more about memory later). As a psychologist, I wonder about the effects of the April 19, 1995, Oklahoma City bombing and the terrorists attacks of September 11, 2001, on babies who were in the womb at that time, especially for those expecting mothers who lost loved ones in either event.

And, oh, my God, what about the peculiar institution called slavery? I digress; that topic is for another day and another book.

2

The Shaping of the Unborn

✦

Pre-birth conditions and attitudes are important to the mom, dad, and fetus, because these are the things that effect the development of the unborn's wombology and sense of self. I developed a variation on Dr. Murray Bowen's (a family therapy pioneer of the 1960s) original genogram, which I call the motherhood genogram, to demonstrate and explain this process. A genogram is a structural or visual diagram that shows multigenerational family relationships and systems. The motherhood genogram consists of at least three generations of women: grandmother, mother, and client if he or she has children. I use this systemic family genogram to show how patterns are transferred from one generation to another and how past events can influence current patterns and family dynamics. The ones involved are usually unaware of what is affecting their daily life.

I love the urban legend that demonstrates generational influences "just because." One Thanksgiving there was three generations of women in the kitchen preparing the dinner—grandmother, mother, and daughter. The mother was just getting ready to cut off the ends of the ham before putting it in the roaster. The daughter asked, "Why are you cutting off the ham like that?" The mother smiled and said, "That's the way my mom did it, so we are passing on the tradition. She turned to Grandma and said, "Right mom?" The grandmother said, "I only did it because the ham was always too big for my small pan. It had nothing to do with tradition." Sometimes traditions have mysterious beginnings, but they become comfortable, easy to follow, and require no extra thinking or questioning. We should wonder why this continues to happen.

If you generate your own motherhood genogram (I explain how to in chapter seven), it will show you where some family dysfunction may have begun, who was challenged by the same things you are, and what you are fighting against without knowing that you are fighting it. After you explore, decode, and gain insight, this motherhood genogram will allow you to use another tool that I learned at a Caroline Myss conference in 2002 called, Call Your Spirit Back (CYSB).[15] It's a way to recognize and acknowledge where you are losing power and energy, and it helps you establish emotional boundaries that help distinguish your emotions from your mother's, to continue the separation process you started on your birthday as you exited your mother's womb.

On the following pages you will see an example of my motherhood genogram. My genogram covers four generations of relationships: my great-grandmother Annie (whom I did not know except through my grandmother), grandmother Nellie (I was 16 when she died), mother Geraldine, and me. You will notice in my genogram a lot of emotional pain connected to births, miscarriages, and children involuntarily released to others' care, all before my mother's wombology experience.

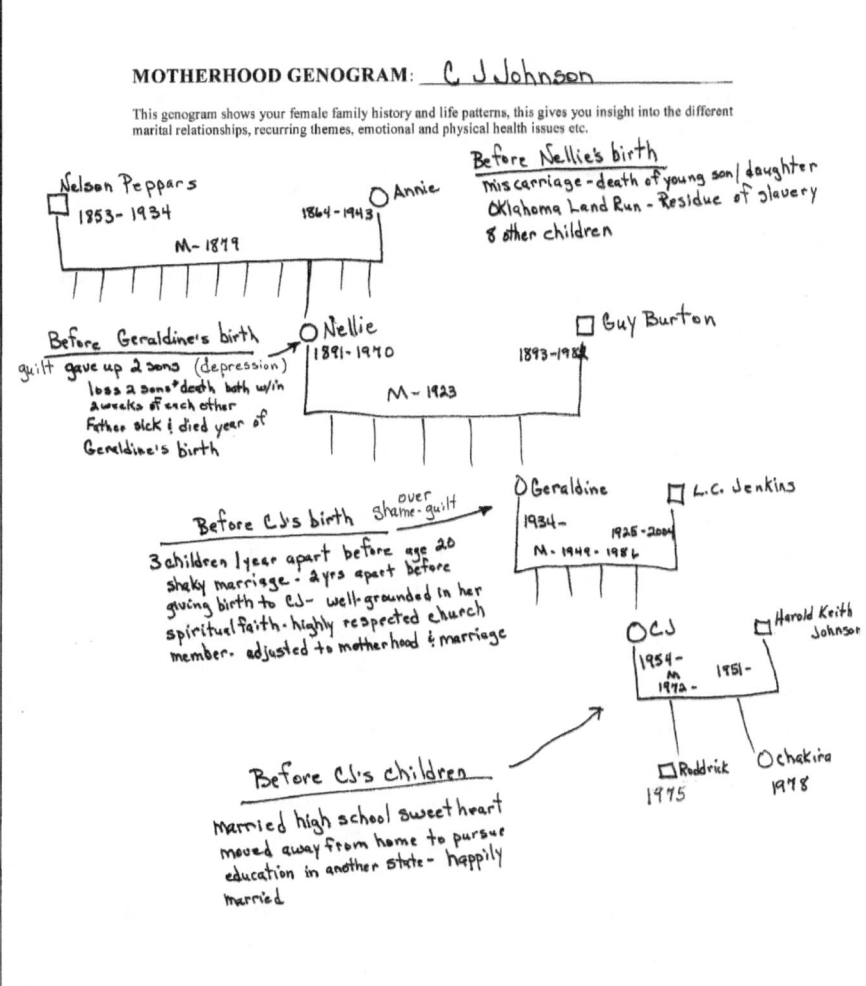

MOTHERHOOD GENOGRAM: C J Johnson

This genogram shows your female family history and life patterns, this gives you insight into the different marital relationships, recurring themes, emotional and physical health issues etc.

Nelson Peppars
1853-1934
M-1879

Annie
1864-1943

Before Nellie's birth
miscarriage-death of young son/daughter
Oklahoma Land Run - Residue of slavery
8 other children

Before Geraldine's birth
guilt gave up 2 sons (depression)
loss 2 sons-death both w/in
2weeks of each other
Father sick & died year of
Geraldine's birth

Nellie
1891-1970
M-1923

Guy Burton
1893-1984

Before CJ's birth shame-guilt over

3 children 1 year apart before age 20
shaky marriage - 2 yrs apart before
giving birth to CJ - well-grounded in her
spiritual faith - highly respected church
member - adjusted to motherhood & marriage

Geraldine
1934-
M-1949-1986

L.C. Jenkins
1925-2004

CJ
1954-
M
1972-

Harold Keith
Johnson
1951-

Before CJ's children

Married high school sweetheart
moved away from home to pursue
education in another state - happily
married

Roddrick
1975

Chakira
1978

Slavery and its residue is a part of my emotional history, as well as unresolved grief over miscarriages and death of children by both Great Grandma Annie and Grandma Nellie. Jeremiah 31:29 discusses the father eating a sour grape, and the children's teeth are set on edge. That same scenario happens with the mothers and is part of my emotional makeup as well.

The recurring emotional theme before me was of guilt, shame, and depression from the unresolved grief and loss issues. The physical theme was and is, "We are strong black women who can handle our trials and tribulations." Each successive generation had smaller families. I'm not sure how many Great-

great Grandma Charity had, but Great Grandma Annie had thirteen children, Grandma Nellie had eleven, Geraldine had four, and I had two. Both of my children are in their thirties and have not started a family.

The zeitgeist for Annie was the Oklahoma Land Run, for Nellie, the Great Depression, and for Geraldine, growing up right after the Great Depression and after her mother had already lost two boys within two weeks of each other to untimely deaths. Even though I did not know these two uncles, who died as teenagers, their deaths' impact on Grandma Nellie had an impact on my mother, which had an impact on me. The impact was on an unconscious level, yet powerful nonetheless.

After I generate a motherhood genogram, I use three books to help establish the zeitgeist before and during the client's utero experience: *The Timetables of History*, by Bernard Grun, *The Century*, by Peter Jennings and Todd Brewster, and *LIFE: Century of Change*, by Richard Stolley, help me use historical information, along with family history, to take a peak at the past and its influence on the future. The concept reminds me of the 1985 movie *Back to the Future*. If you look back, you can often tell your future.

The importance of preexisting attitude, conditions, and environment brings the father into the mix. It goes without saying that the relationship between the mother and the father has a gigantic impact on the mother's emotional state during her pregnancy, which leads to the unborn child's development in the womb spiritually, emotionally, mentally, and physically (SEMP). Dr. Verny presents research that supports the role of the father being more significant than generally accepted.[16] The father's emotional support is essential to the mother's and the unborn child's sense of well-being. We have to lay accountability and responsibility on the father's lap as well as the mother's. Ever since Adam blamed Eve, we mothers get blamed for way too much. If a father is full of anger or resentment because he did not want the pregnancy, and the pregnant woman is constantly afraid of abandonment, that conflict in the relationship has a direct impact on the unborn's wombology. The unborn gets washed in the mother's emotions, which include the chemicals and hormones that accompany emotion, such as cortisol when the mom is stressed, beta-endorphin when pain is present, adrenaline when the mom is frightened or angry, and oxytocin during delivery, which helps wash away the memory of the pain of birth. The unborn child's emotional responses take place long before the limbic system is fully formed (more on that later). If the mother-father relationship is that powerful, it behooves us to pick our baby's dad or mom consciously.

Studies have shown that the unborn child remembers the father's voice too, which allows us to infer that the unborn can detect attitude or mood as well. It does not mean that the fetus can tell when the father is angry, but the effect that anger has on the mother's emotional state is a direct pipeline to the baby's sponge-like emotional state.[17] Can you imagine soaking up all of those emotions and not knowing what to do with them because at this point you are one with Mom? For the unborn, it could feel as if the moods are directed at him. Often babies emerge from the womb wounded and in search of what it takes to make Mom or Dad love, want, and appreciate him in order to finally feel loved. In search of being *good enough* can become a lifetime quest, as Upchurch mentioned. If that approval is not forthcoming, the child can spend a lifetime looking in all the wrong places for something that does not exist or for a substitute. It is difficult to receive love when it was not given to you as a child. Many of my adult clients still believe that they are unlovable and not worthy of a healthy relationship.

Most people who did not get their basic needs met as an infant or child continue to struggle with fear of abandonment, not feeling good enough, or other wombology issues, which keeps the inner child begging for love and attention. Some people are unaware of their wounds because they have always had them, even from the womb, and are therefore not looking for ways to heal their wounds. By the way, just because something is beneath your sense of awareness does not mean that it is not happening or that it does not have an effect on you.

When I taught Psych 101 at a technical college in Griffin, Georgia, and during workshops I give across the nation, we discuss perception and awareness. To demonstrate this point, I usually set out a Color Flow lamp, which continually changes color. When the lights are on in the room, the color change is not detectable; but the minute I turn off the lights, the students and participants are amazed that this lamp was sitting there for two hours emitting color at them and they did not perceive it.

So whether you believe in the inner child concept or not, it affects your daily life. Do you ever wonder why you are afraid to love or be loved? Maybe you are still struggling with inner child issues. Is it difficult to trust yourself or others? Do you have difficulty developing and maintaining healthy relationships? All these issues relate to and could be grounded in your shame-based foundation established in the womb or during early childhood. Most likely some time during in utero, infancy, or childhood, you were left uncovered spiritually, emotionally, and mentally by someone who should have been nurturing and covering you.

My clients who have "trust" issues at different times felt emotionally exposed during childhood and did not experience the nurturing of a mother hen. Part of my purpose on earth is to shine a healing light on this unhealthy darkness and cover those overexposed parts.

When I worked on a chemical dependency unit (CDU) in Colorado, about 88 percent of the female addicts were shame-based and had been molested or sexually abused as a child or preteen, often by a family member or a trusted family friend. Those little girls were left exposed when they should have been covered, protected, and nurtured. The female patients would put themselves down for not being able to get over it and often did not make the connection between their addiction and their wounds. I believe they were trying to soothe their shame-based inner child by feeding her drugs, alcohol, sex, gambling, or other addictions as a replacement for the missing healthy mother's milk. As a child they most likely received toxic mother's milk (symbolically). I witnessed what appeared to be their inner child gagging on all the self-destructive behavior and could hear her cries for help in the form of needing a break from the drugging. Coming in for treatment was the addict's way of shutting up the mind-chatter of the inner child by showing her, "I care enough today to seek help."

An internal battle is usually waged for those struggling with addictions; the mind and the heart are not congruent. The wounded inner child will infuse the adult life with the desire for healing, and when the adult cannot deliver that healing salve, an addiction of some type gets put in the mix of the internal battle. Too many of those clients were the result of an unwanted pregnancy or were survivors of an abortion attempt. Many of them suffered from what I call vaginal fallout syndrome (VFOS), meaning there is no bonding or attachment between mother and child. It is as if the child just fell out of womb or the vagina.

VFOS can start as soon as the infant enters the birth canal to exit the womb, or when the baby peaks its head out of the womb and none of the senses can pick up emotional warmth, such as desire, cherishment, or excitement. It begins at the moment of separation (birth), when the infant exits the womb and is not welcomed into the world by the mother she has been physically connected to for nine months through sounds, food, hormones, and emotional state. Check this list I created to see if you might be dealing with VFOS.

VFOS CHECKLIST

Check these symptoms of VFOS to see if you experience them on a regular basis.

I hate my birthday.
I feel unworthy most of the time.

I have deep-rooted abandonment issues.
Self-destructive behavior is my norm.
I suffer with anxiety disorders.
I have an attachment disorder.
I frequently suffer with depression.

Because of VFOS, many clients have developed misguided habits and behavior that they think are serving them well, so they protect and maintain them. One client told me, "My addiction is my protection. It keeps me safe and acceptable to the outside world. People wouldn't like me if they knew the real me." They often get stuck in the mire of deep-rooted wounds. The best way to heal someone who suffers with VFOS is to help him heal his inner child's memories and become aware of their implicit wounds. It takes time to rebuild character, regulate temperament, and adjust personality, because those deep wounds have always been with that person and he does not know life without the sense of "something is just not right." And too often the person says, "It must be something wrong with me."

John Bradshaw is a delightful gentleman I met at a behavioral science conference. He is a family systems expert and author of many of the books I use for reference during therapy with clients. In his book *Healing the Shame that Binds You*, he discusses healthy shame and toxic shame. Bradshaw writes, "Toxic shame is an excruciating internal experience of unexpected exposure. It is a deep cut felt primarily from the inside. It divides us from ourselves and from others. When our feeling of shame becomes toxic shame, we disown ourselves ... It (shame) loves darkness and secretiveness."[18]

If as a child you were molested (SEMP), you were too young to know about maintaining boundaries, let alone to separate yourself from someone else's stuff. For example, when I was in elementary and middle school, I was often teased or ridiculed about my daddy's illegitimate family. I was embarrassed and took on what should have been the *shhhame* (shhh, keep it a secret) of my father. I was too young to understand that it was not about me. I had no control over my father turning right (to his mistress's house) when he should have turned left (to our house) on the same street. Because of my childhood experiences, I am well acquainted with both forms of shhhame, as well as rejection and ridicule. (I have not forgotten about my own wombology story. I'll get back to it. Promise.)

I must add to Bradshaw's thoughts: this toxic shhhame can indeed begin in the womb and subject you to or expose you to constant anger-shhhame-guilt. And if healthy shame is never modeled or received, your inner child goes on this treacherous journey looking for love in the abyss and is not always successful in finding it.

Toxic shhhame keeps your heart, mood, and mind in the darkness and afraid to reach out to those who want to help you find your way to the light. Your inner child is left crying out or screaming in silence for what I call "eye love," which is that look a loving parent gets in her eyes when she is looking at her bundle of joy, or when one human is so touched by the actions of another that empathy wells up in the person witnessing. Eye love gives the infant the feeling of being cherished, wanted, and loved.

Neuroscientists have discovered the mirror neuron system in the brain. This system allows humans to get deeply involved with others by watching what is happening with others: for example, crying at the movies, screaming at a football game, or laughing with a comic.[19] The addict uses his drug of choice as the pacifier. Just imagine a mother who is struggling with her own inner child's unmet needs during her pregnancy! We have to ask, is that how emotional baggage becomes a generational curse or the start of somatic illnesses that run in the family? This is the type of information we are looking for in the motherhood genogram; it gives us a place to start our journey toward SEMP health.

According to Bradshaw, healthy shame is the structure for modesty, curiosity, creativity, and autonomy, and it safeguards spirituality. I agree and add that these structures are the building blocks for self-esteem, self-acceptance, and self-worth (More on a sense of self in later chapters.) The culture, ethnicity, and era in which we grow feed the shame in our personal growth; they also help determine whether healthy shame or toxic shame is allowed to expand and guide life's path.

Bradshaw informs us, "Healthy shame lets us know that we are limited. It tells us that to be human is to be limited.... Healthy shame is an emotion that teaches us about our limits. Like all emotions, shame moves us to get our basic needs met." Bradshaw shares with us his developmental stages of healthy shame, which is reminiscent of Erik Erikson's psychosocial stages. If you want to know more about Bradshaw's profound and empowering view of the inner child and see his original stages of Healthy (HDL) Shame and Toxic Shame (LDL), pick up a copy of *Healing the Shame that Binds You*.

In Bradshaw's developmental stages of healthy (HDL) shame, the child progresses through five stages. The stages start at age six months and go through adulthood. See the illustration below.

Developmental Stages of Healthy (HDL) Shame

Transcendence   Shame as wisdom, knowing what is valuable and what is not worth your time.

Older Age

Shame as the experience of the Numinous Sacred Holy & Knowing a Higher Power.

Shame as the source and safe guard of spirituality.

Inter-
Dependence   ***Adult***

Experience of life's limits – suffering and death. Shame as knowing you don't know it

all – openness to novelty/creativity.

Young Adult

New secure attachment figure –Love as exposing your vulnerable self. Shame as

modesty.

Independence   ***Puberty***

Shame experienced as limits to self-identity. Shame limits mental curiosity – studiasitas

(temperance of the mind).

Puberty

Emergence of the sex drive experienced as awesome. Healthy shame monitors sex drive.

Shame is dominant in peer group acceptance.

8—Puberty

Shame as Inferiority experienced as limits to one's abilities – social shame related to

ethnicity, gender, status.

8—Puberty

Shame as Embarrassment coming from making mistakes, especially neighborhood social

play –juvenile sex play –social shame as related to belonging.

3.5—8 years

Guilt as moral shame, the internalized parental rules and voices that form conscience.

Early sexual curiosity –manners and modesty.

Counter   ***18 months—3-5 years***
Dependence   Full affect of shame experienced as limits put on child's autonomous need to separate

and do things his or her own way.

6—18 months

Shame as limits to curiosity and interest –when children get into trouble they often hide

their eyes.

Interpersonal	**6 Months**
Bridge	Once securely attached—shame as shyness appears as a
response to being exposed to	
Established	strange faces.
Codependence	

John Bradshaw, figure 1.2 from Healing the Shame That Binds You, Revised and Expanded Edition. Copyright 1988, 2005 by John Bradshaw. Reprinted with the permission of Health Communications, Inc.

If a person does not progress through the stages appropriately, the shame becomes unhealthy or toxic. I believe the foundation for both forms of shame is designed or laid out in the womb during the wombology of a person. I also believe both parents play a huge role in the direction of shame's growth. For example, if the father is not supporting the mother-to-be and is causing her distress, anxiety, or fear, he is contributing to the development of toxic shame by default.

Bradshaw discusses the child hiding his eyes during times of shame, like when he meets a stranger between the ages of six to eighteen months. I find that many adults still avert eye contact or hide their eyes when shame is active, whether it is meeting a stranger or trying to hide or admit to certain types of behavior. My husband has this look down to a perfect science; whenever he gets busted doing something he could have done differently, his head drops, his eyes look down, and his shoulders droop. The kids and I call it his "puppy dog get out of the doghouse" look. It works more often than I want to admit.

I embrace the basic percepts of many original theorists, which means I am an eclectic therapist. My core orientation is Adlerian, which is based on the concepts and theories of Alfred Adler, an Austrian psychiatrist and psychologist and founder of Individual Psychology. My spiritual orientation is based on the theories of Carl G. Jung, a Swiss psychiatrist, psychologist, and founder of what we know as Depth Psychology. Jung is also known for two of my favorite concepts: the collective unconscious and synchronicity, which both support wombology. And I follow Erik H. Erikson, a German Developmental psychologist who is best known for his eight psychosocial stages of development and the phrase "identity crisis." These three psychologists' theories make sense to me and have credibility for me. I use Adler's encouragement theory to empower clients. I use Jung's for clients' spiritual growth. And I use Erikson's stages to show clients possible stages of progression when raising their children or give them a chance to look at their own childhood dysfunction or functionality.

According to stories I've read in historical books on psychology, Erikson was a chauffer for Sigmund Freud (father of psychology) for a while and a friend of Freud's daughter Anna. That might explain why his psychosocial stages are a big contrast to Freud's psychosexual stages. Erikson believed that we develop and progress through eight different psychosocial stages. He emphasized development for a whole lifespan, from infancy to senior citizenship. For our wombology discussion, his first two stages are of main interest. If you want more detailed information on the stages, there are a plethora of books Erikson wrote and books written about his theory of personality development.

Here is my take on his stages and how I use them.

ERIKSON'S STAGES OF PSYCHOSOCIAL DEVELOPMENT

Stage	Conflict	Resolution	
Infancy	Trust vs. mistrust	Find basic sense of trust	Consistent nurturing leads to trust; inconsistent nurturing leads to mistrust
Early childhood	Autonomy vs. shame, doubt	Gain a sense of autonomy	Opportunity to do things for self
Play age	Initiative vs. guilt	Gain a sense of inventiveness	Liberty to play instead of restrictions on every move
School age	Industry vs. inferiority	Learn competency, work ethic	Accomplishments are praised
Adolescence	Identity vs. role confusion	Acquire personal identity	Stable personality in in different situations
Young adult	Intimacy vs. isolation	Find intimate partner	Combining of identity with someone else
Middle age	Generativity vs. stagnation	Concern for future generation	Guiding/helping the next generation
Old age	Integrity vs. despair	Self-acceptance and integration	Being okay with current life situation

My main interest is in Erikson's first two stages of development they show how womb-time can affect the development stages, from infancy to old age. The other stages are self-explanatory and put here so you can see his whole theory. Most theorists agree that early childhood can and most often will influence the whole lifespan. I am suggesting, however, that this influence begins with womb-time, not early childhood. I believe, as Erikson did, that a negative resolution or an unmet need of a stage does not have to cause permanent damage and that the unmet need can be met later in life.

As you can see from the chart above, Erikson's first stage starts with infancy and is concerned with the conflict between trust and mistrust. If an infant learns to trust that his basic needs will be met, he usually grows up as a trusting person and believes the world is trustworthy. But if his needs are not met and mistrust is developed instead, he most likely will grow up believing no one is to be trusted and the world is out to get him. Moving through this stage appropriately or not can predetermine his future view of the world. As an Adlerian psychotherapist, I believe the first recollection becomes the lens through which we view the world; this belief also supports Erikson's first stage view.

Now what if the trust versus mistrust conflict begins in the womb? Don't laugh. Abortion attempt survivors, crack (addict) babies, and other trauma victims have survived a less-than-ideal womb experience. Surely this experience, or lack of trust, colors their future on some level.

Erikson's conflict for the second stage, early childhood, is autonomy versus doubt. In this stage the child is either encouraged or discouraged to separate self from his mom. If Mom encourages autonomy, the child develops confidence in his abilities to do something on his own. But if he is discouraged to discover things on his own, he will begin to doubt his abilities, and a sense of self-doubt sets in. This also is the stage in which I believe the inner child gets wounded most often. (I devote chapter six to the inner child later.) Wombology agrees with Erikson's psychology social stages but proposes that the interaction starts much earlier—as a fetus in the womb instead of during infancy.

I would be neglectful if I ignored Erikson's possible wombology. His biological father was of Danish descent and abandoned Erik's mother while she was pregnant with Erik. This was in Germany, in 1902, and she was Jewish. What do you think her emotional state was for the majority of the time Erik was in the womb? I bet her child's identity was a constant concern for her and later for himself. This might be why he coined the term "identity crisis." The zeitgeist and her culture did not look fondly on a mixing of races. She was a single mother for the first three years of Erik's life before she married his pediatrician. His mom and step-dad kept the details of his biological father and his birth a secret. Think about this: here was this tall, blue-eyed, blond-headed kid who was Jewish. When Erik would go to the temple he was teased about being Nordic, and when he was on the playground at school he was teased for being Jewish. He was the outsider without a real identity, no matter where he was. Maybe that played a huge part in his developing his theory of personality, which focuses on different stages of identity. He was born as Erik Salomonsen, grew up as Erik Homberger, and when he became an American citizen, he officially changed his last name to Erikson—probably in an attempt to finally establish his identity as owning self. Of course, I believe his wombology, which probably included feelings of abandonment and a wounded inner child without an acceptable identity, directed his life path.

If you or someone you love are still coping with abandonment or abuse issues, those issues may very well have started in the womb, so exploring your own wombology is worth the effort to help you move on. Bradshaw warns us,

"All forms of child abuse are abandonment. When parents abuse children, the abuse is about the parent's issues and not the child's. This is why it is abuse."[20] I confirmed what Bradshaw says to be true when I worked on the CD unit, mentioned earlier, in Colorado. I found myself constantly telling the clients, "It's not about you but what happened to you, and now you have to decide whether to nurture the hole in your heart or to nurture a whole heart."

A couple of weeks ago while shopping at a retail superstore, I watched the family dynamics of a mother, father, teenage son, and infant girl. The infant appeared to be about four months old. The father was walking around proudly carrying his daughter, talking and cooing with her, and every now and then the older brother would grasp her little fingers and engage her in coos and conversation. Not once did I see the mother engage with her daughter. I never saw the baby reach out for her or try to get her attention in any way. There was no eye contact between the two, no "eye love." The father would try to engage the mother with the daughter, but she ignored that as well. I watched this in fascination for about thirty-five minutes, as we ended up on the same grocery aisles. At the checkout stand even my husband asked, "Is it my imagination, or has that mother totally ignored that baby throughout the store?" I wanted to go over and hold the baby girl and whisper to her soul, "It's not about you, it's not your fault, and you are worthy." Instead, I invoked a silent prayer that she would grow up joyful in spite of her detached mother. And then I prayed that the mother could heal from her pain. If the mother could heal her pain, it would give the baby girl a better chance of being healthy and to get past her wombology. When the mother in a family system is healthy, the whole family system is healthier, because, as the saying goes, when Mama ain't happy, ain't nobody happy. If the mother-to-be is unhappy, most likely the unborn will be unhappy and has to cope with being unhappy as a newborn.

As I learned from Dr. Northrup, even though this mother may not be engaged or attached to her child, her daughter can physically, at the cellular level, be a part of the mother for up to twenty-seven years after her birth. Dr. Northrup explains, "Recent research has shown that up to seventy percent of pregnant women have fetal cells circulating in their bloodstream by the final trimester of pregnancy. And some have been detected in the circulation of women up to twenty-seven years postpartum!"[21] That is absolutely amazing to me. At the writing of this book, my son is thirty-one years old and my daughter is twenty-eight, which means until recently I could still have some of their fetal cells within my bloodstream. So whether or not we are attached emotionally to our children after giving birth, they may still be physically attached to us.

The emotional attachment and the sense of being cherished, special, and worthy can all happen in an instant, when love is passed from mother to child as their eyes meet. According to Takeo Doi, a psychoanalyst and the author of *The Anatomy of Dependence*, the Japanese have a noun, *amae* (pronounced ah-mah-ay), which means "the expectation to be sweetly and indulgently loved," I don't mean lovingly indulged with material stuff, but to be nurtured and have your needs met, to know when you cry out in pain or hunger someone will come and tend to your needs lovingly.[22] This allows you to move beyond the pain. It starts as a dependent love that we do not outgrow, but its scope changes into interdependent love. If we grow up feeling valued, we can grow through Erikson's developmental stages successfully; if not, we can get stuck at any stage. Many emotional disorders originate with unresolved or unmet childhood needs and unrequited maternal or paternal love. As a result, we continue to look for love in all the wrong places

On the campus where I taught psychology classes, a male student talked with me one day after an emotionally charged class. He had a burning question. "C J, why after thirty-five years do my moms and pops find it so difficult to love me and to understand me?"

My whole body resonated with his desperation and pain. I explained, first of all, that it was not about him. Why was this young man and others like him (Upchurch) going through the futile search for parental love at age thirty-five or older? Often it can be traced back to an Attachment Disorder, a mental and emotional condition that occurs in the first three years of development, where the child does not attach, bond, or trust his mother or caregiver. It becomes difficult for the child to get his needs met. If a mother and child have a relationship that is close, secure, and *amae*, the child learns to generalize trust, love, and security during his lifespan. If the relationship is detached and distant, the child generalizes that, too, over a lifespan. Many times adopted and foster care children struggle with attachment disorders, specifically Reactive Attachment Disorder (RAD), but the struggle also can come from a birth mom who is so self-absorbed that it is difficult for her to nurture anyone other than herself. If you had a mother who was challenged by Borderline Personality Disorder (BPD) or clinical depression, you may know exactly what I'm saying.

John Bowlby, a British psychoanalyst who is considered the father of Attachment Theory, believed that attachment begins at infancy and continues throughout the lifespan. It is assumed that the attachment behaviors an infant develops will help shape attachment relationships he has as an adult.[23] Dr. Mary Ainsworth, a partner of Bowlby and mother of the Strange Situation attachment model, used three types of attachment when studying the interactions between mother and child when they have been separated and reunited. Ainsworth used Bowlby's model as her foundation. The three types—secure, avoidant, and resistant—explain the mother-child relationship. The secure type is when the infant looks for comfort from her mother and receives nurturing consistently. The mother is usually considered to be loving and affectionate. The avoidant type is when the infant tends to ignore the mother or pull away from her. The mother is usually considered detached or rejecting of the infant's attachment behavior. The resistant type is when the infant clings to his mother. The mother is usually considered to be inconsistent in her care. This mother-child attachment bond type influences other relationships through out a life time.[24]

I agree with both of their models about the importance of the attachment relationship happening as soon as possible after birth and that the attachment influences a lifetime of relationships. But I believe that mother-child and father-child bonds of attachment must start with the attitude of the parents while the infant is in the womb. If the bond never takes place, usually a family system struggles with attachment drama, behavioral problems from the children, and SEMP burnout from the parents (caregivers).

What if emotional attachment disorder begins in the womb with an unsuccessful abortion attempt? I have had many clients who were in their fifties and still struggling with mother-daughter issues. Their mothers told them that she either considered abortion or attempted it. That disclosure played on the heart and soul of my clients. Now why would a mother tell her child that injurious fact? I don't know.

When I was researching topics for this book, I communicated with Dr. Verny via e-mail and asked him if there were any statistics on abortion attempt survivors. He directed me to many of the studies, Web sites, and literature on those people who have survived abortion attempts. If you put the words *abortion survivor* in your favorite search engine, you will be amazed at the stories that jump out at you! Before writing this book, I never thought about how many abortion survivors who might be struggling with attachment issues. Some of their pain could be from a failed abortion, and they do not know that.

Sometimes I ask clients to tell me a story about any part of their childhood, a part of therapy I call The Legend of You. The following story is what one client, Ganci, shared with me.

> Once upon a time, in a vision, I saw a little girl crouched in a corner of what looked like a cave. Her hands were tightly covering her eyes, and she was in a tensed, curled position. She didn't move from the curled position, nor would she uncover her eyes. To her, all was dark, silent, and lonely. She never uttered a word, changed her position, or uncovered her eyed as long as I was watching.

As I watched, I began to see a bigger picture. Light was all around the area of the little girl, but because of her hands she couldn't see the light. Jesus was also within the light. (No, I didn't actually see him, but I could sense he was in the midst of the light.) I could sense the little girl in the cave wanted to change her position and uncover her eyes, but she was afraid. She was afraid that if she did, she would get hurt again. She was afraid that if she did, she would get abused again and she would feel worse than she already did.

Then the truth came to me: I was that little girl in the cave! It was I who was curled in the fetal position, hands covering my eyes and afraid to move. It was I who was afraid to move, hoping that if I didn't move I could not be hurt again. Then I realized … only I could remove my hands from my face, only I could change my position, and only I could leave the cave …"

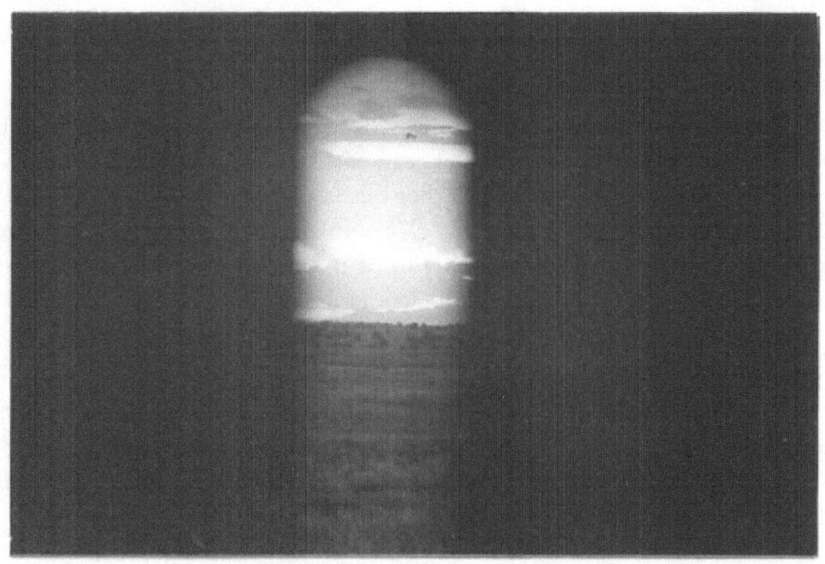

Looking out from inside the cave

If we use symbolic insight to interpret Ganci's story, the cave is her mother's womb, and knowing that only she could change positions or leave the cave represents the birth canal. The attacks she feared would continue were abortion attempts. The self-defense and tightened fetal positions indicate survival mode. Ganci was the fifth and last child, with five years between her and her next sibling. Their mother suffered from major depression disorder, and Ganci was told often as a child by her parents and siblings that she was an unwanted pregnancy. Today, Ganci still battles depression, low self-esteem, low self-worth, and abandonment issues. She had used drugs as her pacifier and love replacement for thirty years before we met.

For many women, self-inflicted abortions were the solution to unwanted pregnancies, especially before abortion was legalized. What if failure to thrive or attachment disorders are the baby's response to abortion attempts that the mother has never disclosed? It would be most difficult to attach or bond to someone who you feel on a primal level has tried to take your life. If that is true, I wonder how many people never have been able to bond with their biological mother, even though she has been there and given her best. Do these people now deal with on a primordial level survivor's guilt, victim's anger, or an unconscious, deep-felt sense that there is something wrong with them because an attempt on their life took place in the womb?

In *The Secret Life of the Unborn Child*, Dr. Verny discusses the lack of bonding between a mother and child in chapter three. At birth, this infant was healthy and full of life. Then for some reason the baby would not move toward her mother's breast. Each time the mother offered her breast, the baby would reject it and turn the other way. This scenario played out for several days before the attending doctor devised an experiment. Another nursing mother offered her breast to the infant; instead of rejecting this stranger's breast, the infant began sucking for her life.

The doctor asked the mother, "Why do you suppose the child reacted that way?" The woman had no clue until the doctor asked her, "Well, did you want to get pregnant then?" The woman said, "No, I didn't. I wanted an abortion. My husband wanted the child. That's why I had her."[25] On a soul level the baby already knew this.

For women who have struggled with the pain of miscarriage, stillborn babies, and crib death, I believe the soul of the baby you carried decided for whatever reason that it was not ready or willing to come to earth and changed its mind and went back to its original comfort zone. Unless you were purposely injurious to yourself or the baby in hopes of helping it exit your womb, it was not so much what you did or did not do to make it happen. It was not your fault that the soul simply decided not yet, which had nothing to do with you as a vessel to get it here. It does not mean you are not worthy; the soul decided that it was not ready for this earthly journey.

For the women I have counseled who found themselves going through the difficult decision, grief, loss, and secrecy of an abortion, it was usually a choice she wished she did not have to make. There are so many recorded cases of babies surviving abortion attempts that I believe if a soul is ready to come to earth, mankind cannot stop it.

If you went through this experience or are a survivor of this ordeal, I hope something in this book resonates with you and you can find some resolution for the pain you may still be suffering so that you can heal and continue your personal growth. You might be able to help others who have gone through similar circumstances. It is a part of the past that cannot be changed.

A healthy happy baby is a priceless gift worth giving to the whole family and society. I tell my clients with children, "You are not raising little boys or little girls. You are raising men and women. What you do or don't put in them can last a lifetime." Implicit messages can be more damaging than explicit ones. Remember, the unborn is not savvy enough yet to discern where the line of separation begins or ends. You do not want to be responsible for the neoteny, or arrested development, of your children.

(Speaking of arrested development, I wonder what some of the troubled entertainers who are always in the news for some misguided or self-destructive behavior received in the womb.)

Abbey, another ex-client who is an adoptee, was able to generate conversations when I asked her to imagine being in the womb and tell me what surfaced for her. On the following page you can explore what Abbey generated when she imagined her wombology story. I am grateful to her for letting me share it with you. We used symbolism and knowledge of her pre-birth environment to determine that she witnessed conversations between her biological mother, biological grandmother, and biological father.

While her mother was pregnant with Abbey, her husband was having an affair with her own mother. Did you get that one? It took me a while. Abbey's biological father was having an affair with her biological grandmother while her mother was pregnant with her. Whew! Talk about grandmother-daughter issues! This is what broke up the marriage and was the reason Abbey was adopted. Gail and Chuck, (Abbey's bio-parents) already had two children together, but Gail could not handle having a constant reminder of her own mother's and husband's betrayal, so she gave Abbey up for adoption. Abandonment and unworthiness were a constant emotional state for Gail while pregnant. And the question, "What is so wrong with me that my husband of nine years would leave me pregnant and alone for my own mother?" ruminated through her whole being.

Abbey was born in the South, but her adoptive parents lived and raised her in Mormon territory. Abbey spent most of her life trying to fit into a family and community that didn't fit her original environment, and as a teen she developed BPD. She is now in her early thirties and has finally come to terms with her original environment. She has outgrown many of her borderline tendencies.

Can you imagine what she received in the womb and how alienated she must have felt most of her childhood and teen life?

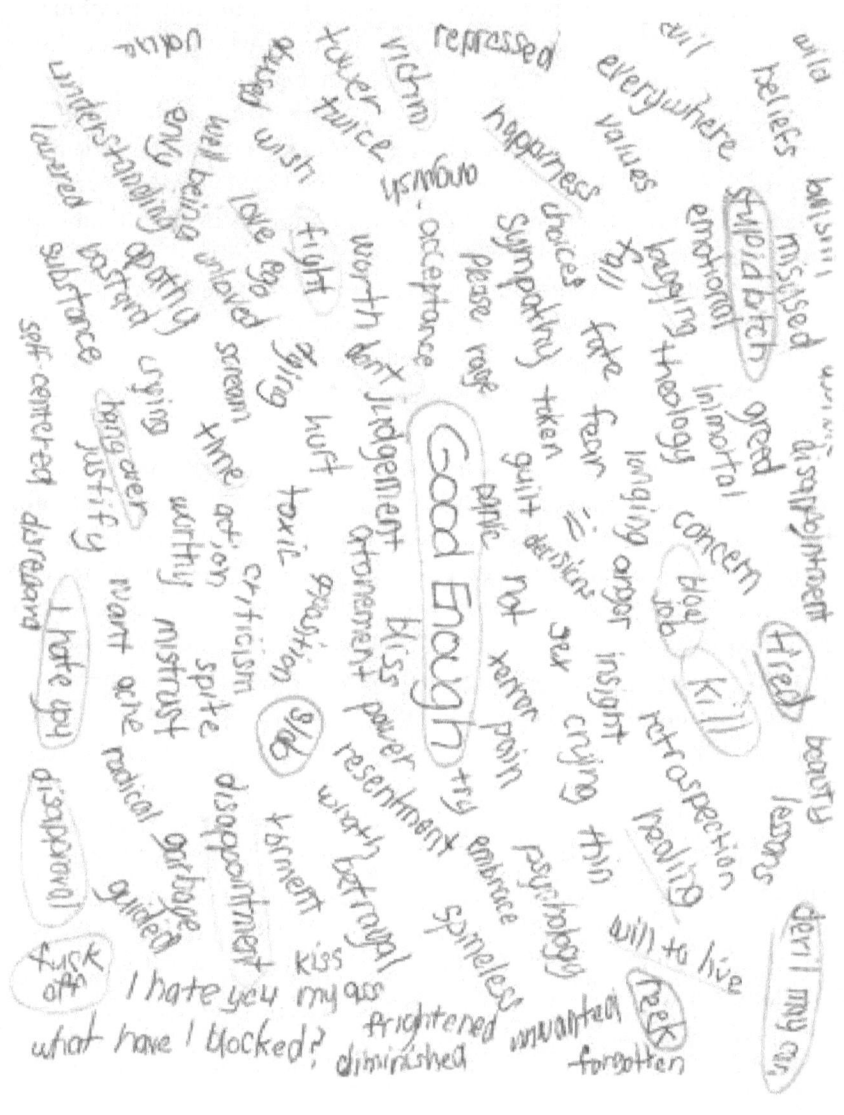

Abbey's voices

3

Angry All the Time

✦

I am an avid yard-dog (gardener). One day while working in my front yard, a guy driving a van stopped and said, "I love to see someone who enjoys taking care of his or her yard. I enjoy what I do too. It plays into what you are doing. I pressure-wash houses for cheap." He chuckled and said, "Actually, I spent too much money this past weekend while drinking and pretending to be someone I'm not, so I have to make up the money spent. Do you want your house pressure-washed?"

As a psychologist, I could not resist asking who was he pretending to be, and that started us on a ninety-minute conversation in which he (Donald) shared many of his life's questions and struggles. When he found out I was a psychologist he said, "If you can fix me, I'll do your house for cheaper than cheap."

About forty minutes into the conversation I explained wombology. His mouth flew open and his eyes bugged out as he said, "Oh, my God, that explains so much that I couldn't get from my bible," (Scott Peck's *A Road Less Traveled*), which he showed me. It was tattered from use. Then he said, "C J, I feel in my heart that I am kind and easygoing, but instead I am quick to anger, slow to forgive, and blame others for my problems." That is when I asked him if he knew anything about his mom's emotional state when she was pregnant with him. Turns out she was angry all the time because they lived the military life and she was not able to stay near her mother during her first pregnancy.

The most difficult FOOLISH ghost dance to dislodge from the body and mind is the stored misperception of being unworthy. It is the number one challenge for 90 percent of my clients, especially for the domestic violence victims I worked with for four years. It was helpful when we could solve their private mystery through their wombology story. Once the pain-filled memories become *just a story*, wombology issues no longer hold the emotional electricity that they did previously. With each experience of telling or processing her story, the person moved closer to emotional freedom.

If you have unresolved wombology or inner child issues, you will find yourself being impatient, irritated, and frustrated when someone else's inner child cries out for help. It is almost impossible to understand, empathize, or accept someone else's feelings, positive or negative, if your own "stuff" has not been heard, validated, or witnessed. Healing your negative feelings from the past is imperative for your future and your loved ones, including those you do not even know yet! Every morning in my prayers I pray for all my loved ones and others who will cross my path, including those I do not know yet, such as grandchildren, new clients, or a person I might meet at a workshop who becomes a friend.

In his book *Men Are from Mars, Women Are from Venus*, John Gray tells us that if our past were different, we would be different. If we were exposed to mutually loving relationship between our parents, we can love and communicate not just our love, but our hurt or negative feelings without discounting the other person.[26] But since most of us were not that blessed, we have to develop enough self-trust, self-love, and self-confidence to be able to communicate honesty without a hidden agenda. At any point in your life you can only give what you currently have. If you have a heart filled with joy, you will give others joy. If you are filled with anger, you will give away anger. That is just how it works. Pepsi cannot give you the taste of Coca-Cola or vice versa!

On the following pages are three checklists to help you assess your anger awareness and to help you figure out whether it is yours or not. The first one, "Checklist of Hidden Anger," is an example of how many people express suppressed anger. (I developed this checklist from a combination of anger management tools I have used over the years.) Do you have insidious behaviors (check out numbers 2, 3, and 12 of the checklist) that you keep ignoring? Is this behavior below your sense of awareness? The checklist contains eighteen indicators; if you check four, you need to explore the source of your anger. If you check nine or more, get to an anger awareness workshop fast.

One prospective client was so full of anger that when I asked him to consider breathing deeply instead of raging or to practice patience and tolerance toward his siblings, he decided I was not the psychotherapist for him—although he admitted that his FOO (family of origin) and many girlfriends had told him to get some help with his anger issues. In addition, he had spent two years inside a federal "gated community" (penitentiary) for an angry outburst at his workplace. He kept insisting through clenched jaws, "I don't have anger issues, and I'm sick and tired of people telling me that I do." Hmmm. If complete strangers notice you seem angry, you just might want to check it out from someone else's point of view. Some people are completely unaware of how others experience them. The Johari Window is an excellent tool to help you see another's perception of you (more on that in chapter seven).

The second checklist, "Growing Up in an Angry House," which I developed while managing the battered women's shelter, has examples of what can happen when a person grows up in a house full of anger, hidden or overt. Many children of alcoholics have experienced these examples and have learned what to do or not do. There are nine indicators; check all that apply. If you check four or more, it is time to explore how anger plays out in your daily life. These examples help you decide who is in control of your emotions—you or your past. If you decide it is your past, take the time to discover whose anger is directing your current life. When you were growing up, were you allowed to express your emotions (anger)? Even though I was probably the most vocal of Mom's four children (babies often are), I still had to be very careful with verbalizing my emotions. I remember once my dad slapped me because he thought I was talking back, and, of course, I wasn't talking back. To him, talking back was a huge sign of disrespect, and he was not having any of that, baby girl or not. If you were not allowed to express your emotions, you usually learned how to suppress them in order to survive or gain the approval of your caretakers.

Anger is often a cover-up for emotions you are afraid to share or express. Beneath the cloak of anger is usually a fear of losing something or someone. The third checklist, "Anger's Secret Dozen," addresses this. I developed it while working with the victims of domestic violence. It assesses what you are too timid to share with others. Picture an iceberg with anger being the part that is visible above the water's surface and the secret dozen list as the massive, unseen, dangerous foundation lying beneath the surface. "Out of sight, out of mind" does not mean if it is below your sense of awareness that it is not directing your daily life. Check off all that apply of the secret dozen that you experience weekly or daily. If you check three or more, it is time to find someone you trust who will help you dig deep enough to move beyond the grip of "Anger's Secret Dozen."

CHECKLIST FOR HIDDEN ANGER

Here is a checklist to help you determine if you are hiding your anger, even from yourself, and if your inner child is controlling most of your day. Any of these is usually a sign of unresolved and hidden anger.

- ❏ **"Clenched jaws" (TMJ) – especially while sleeping – too angry to talk**

- ❏ **Procrastination in the completion of agreed upon tasks**

- ❏ **Like to use sadistic humor**

- ❏ **Irritable bowel syndrome – can't let go or won't let go – fear of losing**

- ❏ **Excessive sleepiness – don't want to deal with the real world**

- ❏ **Stiff neck or sore shoulders – carrying too heavy a load**

- ❏ **Chronically depressed without a cause**

- ❏ **Fist clenching while talking**

- ❏ **Going off over the little things – being overlooked again**

- ❏ **Smiling through the pain – if I keep smiling no one will know**

- ❏ **Recurring nightmares – your boogeyman won't let go of you**

- ❏ **Habitually late – wait for me if you really care**

- ❏ **Always polite – let me take care of you**

- ❏ **Frequent sighing or holding your breath – afraid to take** a deep breath

❑ Use of sarcastic remarks – flippant in conversations

❑ Monotone voice (Ben Stein) – don't show emotions

❑ Easily bored

❑ Apathetic toward others

This checklist is not about obvious rage. This is about those little things you do but probably unaware that you do them. Could this be your inner child throwing yet another temper tantrum? If you checked seven or more of the above items you need to work on your hidden anger.

Did growing up in an angry house teach you how to...?

Check all that apply.

❑ **Hide your emotions**

❑ **Hide yourself**

❑ **Self-medicate (addictions)**

❑ **Bob and weave continuously**

❑ **Be evasive**

❑ **Avoid life**

❑ **Lie to protect...**

❑ **Survive, not thrive**

Anger is usually the effect of crossed boundaries. If you checked three or more, it is time to work on the root cause of your anger, which could have started during your womb time.

Checklist for Anger's Secret Dozen

Check all that apply.

- ☐ **Abandonment**

- ☐ **Dependency**

- ☐ **Depression**

- ☐ **Fear**

- ☐ **Frustration**

- ☐ **Guilt**

- ☐ **Hurt**

- ☐ **Mistrust**

- ☐ **Powerlessness**

- ☐ **Rejection**

- ☐ **Shame**

- ☐ **Unlovable**

If you have constantly been challenged by three or more of these anger-based issues and don't know why, it is time to explore your wombology. Awareness is the first step toward healing.

Abraham H. Maslow was a humanistic psychologist who developed a motivational theory (check it out below) that emphasized why a person would strive to reach their full potential or become self-actualized. Maslow's hierarchy of needs purported that if the lower needs are met, the higher needs can be attained and influence our behavior.[27] His theory meets my theory on unexpressed or unresolved anger on the second tier, where you can get stuck no matter what your social economic status might be.

Let's say you have your basic biological and physiological needs met, which consist of air, food, water, shelter, sleep, and sex. But safety needs of protection, security, order, and stability are not met. You might use an angry demeanor as a way to keep people from getting too close to you emotionally, so it becomes a form of protection. The cloak of anger becomes your security blanket, as with the prospective client I mentioned before. Anger can even help you keep things in order. Think about it. How fast can you clean your kitchen if you are angry compared to when you're happy or sad? I can hear your cabinet doors slamming and the pots clanging right now. When my mom gets upset or angry, she will get a broom and become the sweeping machine; every floor in the house gets swept, carpeted or not. Zora Neale Hurston, a folklorist and writer during the Harlem Renaissance, said, "Grab the broom of anger and drive off the beast of fear."[28] I'm not the only one who knows anger gives you energy and physical power.

If you did not get your safety needs met in childhood, it becomes more challenging for you to let go of that need to fill that void or to let go of the FOOLISH ghost dance. When you focus on what you did not get or do not have, you find a way to stay locked or stuck in a "mode of lacking" mentality. Too many of my clients live in their head, which often means wallowing in the pain for something that happened in the past instead of living in the now. We all live at our mental address, which means that what we focus on becomes our daily life. If you choose to stay angry and in stage two, getting to stage five (personal and spiritual growth) will not happen. Again, if you needed Pepsi and received Coca-Cola, you may still feel cheated out of what was rightfully yours. In reality, there is a life force within all of us that drives us to seek and reach for more, but if you continue to suppress it with righteous anger, the iceberg's foundation gets deeper and larger and harder to reach. Anger awareness, whether it comes from wombology or current events, gives you more control of relationships.

Maslow's Hierarchy of Needs

STAGE FIVE
Self-actualization
Spiritual and personal growth

STAGE FOUR
Esteem needs
Achievements, status, reputation

STAGE THREE
Belonging and love
Family, social acceptance, affection

STAGE TWO
Safety needs
Protection, security, order, stability

STAGE ONE
Biological and physiological needs
Basic life-giving needs: food, water, air, shelter, warmth

Once you comprehend and accept that some of your anger issues are part of your wombology story or understand that wombology is something that happened to you but is not who you have to be for the rest of your life, the transformation to being who you truly are begins. And that transformational journey can begin with learning to reframe your personal story. In order to become unchained from your unnamed pain or anger, you may have to reframe the way it first came—and maybe it is a parent's unclaimed anger or pain. For instance, when I reframed my childhood relationship with my father, who was a detached father, my childhood longing was given freedom or wings. You can read my reframed story in the Appendix. Remember, your story is not a part of your DNA, which means you can let go of your woundology and wombology. It's your choice.

In one of my favorite daily meditation books, *The Soul's Companion*, by author Dr. Tian Dayton, she gives us permission to not accept our roles as our full or only identity: "I am more than my roles."[29] I love that quote. We are more than the angry daughter/son, mother/father, sister/brother. Even if you chose your role, it does not mean you have to play that role forever. Our walk on earth is about growing spiritually, not getting stuck in one character.

Once you realize it's not about you but what happened to you, you move closer to living fully and growing through your experiences. I have a client who does not accept that she deserves love, recognition, cherishment, or validation. "If I didn't get it from my family, why should I expect it now? Why couldn't they show me love then? Not once did my parents tell me that they loved me and was glad I'm here." When I try to convince her of her worth as a special, gifted person, she looks at me as if I'm blind or conning her. Three years later it is still difficult for her to receive those words as truth.

This is yet another reason to unravel the entanglement with what you received in the womb. Through the unraveling process, your perception of reality can change. If you grew up in that angry house, it is difficult to get hurtful words out of your head; but don't stay stuck in that house … get into your life instead.

What if your personal wombology story becomes just that—your story of what happened, not what is still happening? Of course, some people are so attached to their wounds and body-based memories that they continue to re-traumatize themselves again and again. Those are the people who *do not* want to heal.

One of the biggest "aha" moments for me was when I finally understood that there are people who refuse to get better, to let go of their past, and who will not disconnect from their umbilical cord of anger's pain. Status quo is their comfort zone, and anger's pain is their constant companion. And for some, it is a reminder that they are actually alive. My higher learning did not teach me that one; I learned it through my clinical experience. When I recognize that a client is practicing what Caroline Myss, intuitive healer and author of *Anatomy of the Spirit*, calls woundology (an exchange of wound stories that take over a conversation and sometimes used to bind a relationship), I refer them to someone else.[30] If I continued with a client who is practicing woundology, therapy would become sessions of venting and whining, not psychotherapy, because that person is not ready for personal growth. Thanks, but no thanks; I'll pass on that one. That's not to say we all do not vent or whine at times, but if that is all you do at each session, it is not therapeutic and does not foster personal growth. Unresolved anger prevents you from healing because you cannot heal what you refuse to feel.

The following quote sums up what I mean about people not wanting to grow beyond their pain, no matter how old the original event might be or how long they may live.

"People have a hard time letting go of their suffering. Out of fear of the unknown, they prefer suffering that is familiar." —Thich Nhat Hanh, Buddhist monk

4

Mind over Matter: What's in the Mind Matters

✦

Bear with me while I veer into the scientific realm. To fully understand the many implications of wombology, we first need to grasp the mental, somatic, and emotional connection through neuropsychology, which is the study of the relationship between the brain's functions, our emotions, and behavior. This discipline of psychology overlaps with neuroscience, philosophy, neurology, and psychiatry. In layman's terms, neuropsychology aims to clarify and explain the relationship between what we think, feel, and do.

I will not go into a deep explanation of the difference between the brain and the mind, but I will say the brain weighs approximately three pounds and has limits, whereas the mind is weightless and limitless. The mind uses cognition as the process to gain knowledge or become aware of events or objects in our environment, and then we use that knowledge for comprehension and problem solving. The cerebral cortex is the outermost layer of the cerebral hemispheres of the brain. It is largely responsible for all forms of conscious experience, including perception, emotion, thought, and planning—in other words, cognition. Our mind is what separates us from our family in the animal kingdom.

The brain has three main parts: the forebrain, midbrain, and hindbrain. The part of the brain that we are concerned with is the forebrain. It contains the limbic system, which is a group of brain structures that includes the amygdala, hippocampus, and other structures that regulate the expression of emotions, how we receive emotion, and emotional memory.

According to Philip G. Zimbardo et al., in the textbook *Psychology Core Concepts*,[31] "Emotion is a state of mental and physical arousal focused on some event or situation of importance to the person. Emotions help us respond to our world and convey to others our intentions usually through our behavior."

The adage "actions speak louder than words" comes alive in this description of emotions. Two distinct systems in the brain are involved in the physical responses of cognition (limbic) and the feelings of emotion (amygdala).

The limbic system is considered the emotion pathway. The amygdala is an almond-shaped structure in the forebrain that plays a central role in emotional learning, especially within the context of fear. It receives messages from both the implicit (something not deliberately learned or of which you have no conscious awareness) and explicit (something that has been processed with your attention and can be consciously recalled) pathways and helps attach meaning to our emotions. It is more involved with the unconscious or implicit levels of processing of what we experience. The hippocampus is a seahorse-shaped structure that helps with learning, memory, and emotions.

The cerebral cortex is involved with the conscious, or explicit level, of processing those things we experience.

The cerebral hemispheres are the two halves of the brain. The two hemispheres play their own role in regulating emotions. I'm sure that you have heard of people discussing whether they are right-brained or left-brained. It is a simplistic way to proclaim what they feel is their most dominant hemisphere when they deal with daily life. The right brain's processing is more visual, spatial, symbolic, creative, and aesthetic. In comparison, the left-brain's processes are more analytical, linear, logical, and rational. For instance, I joke about being so right-brained that I can't see left. And my daughter often says, "Mom, try using the left side of your brain today." She is considered left-brain dominant, which could explain why she is a great civil engineer. My left-brainlessness could explain why I am great in psychology. Often mentally we are worlds apart, but our separateness helps each one of us stay well-rounded. (Now, how I had a left-brained child is another mystery for another day. Oops, mystery solved: her father is left-brained. I imagine that he had a part to play in her genetics! I'll write more on how I make myself a little more whole-brained later.) Leonardo da Vinci is my favorite whole-brained person. He probably was one of those people who used all parts of his brain.

The left hemisphere of the brain specializes in positive and joyful emotions.[32] The right hemisphere of the brain specializes in negative emotions, like anger and depression. This split is called lateralization of emotions, discovered by researchers studying people who had damaged that area of the brain. When you look at this lateralization symbolically it makes sense, because the left side of the body represents the feminine side of us, and the right side of the body represents the masculine side of us. And in our society it is expected for the woman to be positive and joyful, to be the nurturer, while society requires that the man be the protector, using anger as a tool to disguise his fear and depression. He is expected to protect or fix everything.

Why are we concerned with all of this brain and mind data, when it is the heart that gets broken or is considered the seat of the soul? Because the brain is the director, even though the mind is the master, of what we experience through our perception and biology. Even though the brain only weighs about three pounds, it holds tons of emotions, memories, habits, and characteristics via the mind. If a person resides in your head, he or she is never dead. Our body often speaks the mind by manifesting different discomforts that affect our health and emotions. The mind is like the technician who guides the pilot of an airplane with special flashlights signaling to the pilot which way to turn the wheels in order to safely park at the terminal. I hope you use this book and its contents as the person with the light directing you to a safe landing. If you want to change your life, you have to change your mind first. Sometimes in the flow of life we need someone to guide us to a safe place to park.

In their book *Mind, Body, Spirit: Connecting with Your Creative Self,* authors Mary Braheny and Diane Halperin write, "The body is an incredible mechanism and has an astonishing memory; it never forgets. Muscle groups compensate for each other and unexpressed feelings as well as trauma are stored in tissue, waiting for a time to come to the surface."[33] If we accept this as truth, and I do, does that mean we can come into this world with somatic memory capsules (cell memory) or suffering from the symptoms of Posttraumatic Stress Disorder (PTSD) from the trauma received in the womb? Oxytocin is the hormone released into the bloodstream during labor, and it can help erase the memory of the pain of giving birth and of being born from the mind, but maybe not from the body.

Imagine the things some people received in the womb. As they try to progress through Erikson's or Bradshaw's stages, they are considered sensitive or difficult babies, when in reality they may be on some level experiencing some primordial memory, flashback, or somatic reenactment of a traumatic experience in utero.

Could wombology explain the difference between a sensitive and calm baby?

You cannot heal what you cannot feel

5

Healing Memories

✦

Memory is commonly defined as the cognitive or information-processing system that encodes (gathers), stores, and retrieves information.

There are three main stages of memory. Sensory memory (SM) uses our five senses to gather and hold information briefly. It lasts about one-fourth of a second. Short-term memory (STM) uses the hippocampus to gather information, add meaning to it, and make it acceptable for long-term storage. It lasts for about thirty seconds. Long-term memory (LTM) has a large capacity to store material organized by its meaning. The duration and storage capacity with LTM are unlimited.

There are numerous types of memories—implicit memory—material, events, situations of which we have no conscious awareness but can affect our emotions and behavior; explicit memory—material, events, situations that we are aware of that also can affect our emotions and behavior; flashbulb memory—a clear and vivid long-term memory of an especially meaningful and emotional event (such as the Oklahoma City bombing in 1995); and episodic memory—personal events or episodes (such as your first kiss).

Why are we going through the structure and functions of memory? Because our memory of an event or situation keeps us hurting or re-injuring ourselves, not the event. According to the definitions proposed, wombology deals with implicit memories. The body never forgetting explains why emotional memories are the hardest to release, since we receive them through our sensory pathway. For example, the sense of smell is one of the quickest routes to memory lane. Think about how a certain aroma of food or perfume can instantly make you remember a person, place, or event.

Braheny and Halperin write about infants, "Through images and sensory impressions the infant absorbs an awareness of himself and of how to survive through a world of picture and tactile/kinesthetic impressions. Family dynamics are perceived and felt as images that are stored in the body and used as information on how to interact in the family…. Residual tensions in body parts contain the family secrets."[34] Verny adds, "Much of what a newborn learns in the first days of life, he learns through his eyes…. Eyes tell him a lot, but touch tells him even more. Stroking, petting, and holding are an infant's information source—a way of making some important judgment about the other person…. If an infant is approached in a cool, disinterested, suffocating or angry manner it tells him he is unloved and perhaps, even in some danger."[35] Your preverbal development gives you your first impressions and perceptions of your family dynamics and how the family experiences you: good, bad, or indifferent. We use all of our senses before and after birth to explore our environment and other people's feelings toward us.

Family secrets gets lodged as cell memories in the body, and if you don't resolve those childhood wounds, you will continue to manifest your own form of chaos or play out the family untruths through the FOOLISH ghost dance.

The body never forgets. One day while picking wild plums in the countryside with Mom, Aunt Geneva, and Linda, I spotted what I thought was a beautiful native plant. I wanted to take some of it home to Georgia to plant, but Aunt Geneva shuttered and said, "Guhl, don't take that mess. That is ironweed, and I got a many of whippings with it. I can still feel the sting on my legs." Aunt Geneva was eighty at the time of our outing, and she was recalling whippings from seventy-five years earlier.

Wombology and inner child work is intimate, deep, and power-filled. It is essential that you create a SEMP safe space and place to do your inner healing work. Emotional freedom is yours if you are ready and willing to do the work. Hopefully, through this book you are learning what it takes to be aware, awake, and alert and how to use those things to live consciously and purposefully. Do not be a self-help book junkie, meaning you read as many self-help books as possible, but after reading the material you put the book on a shelf and go about your life the same as you did before reading it. In the words of a wise elderly woman from my hometown, " Honey, once you wake up, don't go back to sleep." You have to stay awake because you now know that you are responsible for seven generations. Your choices and decisions will have a direct impact on your seven. I promise this to be a truth.

Your voice can abort or give birth to something new daily. Why not start with a new you? For me, voice equals choice. Now is the time to give voice to your symbolic womb and allow its healing. You cannot force healing; you have to allow it to happen. For most of us, it does not happen in an instant. If you will get rid of your misery, you will not pass it down as a mystery to your child or grandchild. Remember, unresolved emotions can become generational, especially with depression and anger as the foundation.

In order to recover and release the trauma placed within your psyche in utero, whether by your grandmother's daughter or your father, give yourself time and space to explore your wombology. Just remember that you are processing someone else's "stuff," removing it from your psyche. Try this exercise: put yourself in your mother's space (SEMP) when she was carrying you—as if it were you in the exact time (1953, for instance), situation (black woman in rural Oklahoma), and place emotionally (happy). What would you have done differently? For this exercise I use the timeline books I mentioned before. It is different when you see events from the eyes of history. Write down your responses and reactions in your journal. As you do this intimate work, please do not judge yourself or your parents; just feel your emotions fully and release what is not helping you to grow. No judgments; just exploration of who you are. Remember, it is not about you but about what happened to you.

Some of us were blessed enough to receive more positive than negative states and do not have to struggle with discerning what is ours and what is our parents'. We are okay with our characteristics, personality traits, and temperament and do not have to work to compensate for our wombology. Socrates said, "The unexamined life is not worth living."[36] I agree, of course, and think there is still need to examine the different aspects of ourselves (SEMP). Whether your first environment was negative or positive, being aware of it can improve our understanding of who we are today. Armed with self-knowledge about our dark side (shadow) and light side, our wombology story, and a healthy inner child, we can help others find the unshakable serenity and joy we possess.

On February 5, 1998, at 5:00 PM as I was reading John Gray's book *Men Are from Mars, Women Are from Venus,* I received a full vision of my purpose, which is to help others heal from their grief and loss issues by helping them reduce their emotional pain. I now realize we have *purposes*—not just one purpose—and part of that purpose includes taking care of seven generations. Dr. Christiane Northrup tells us that when we heal ourselves today, our ancestors can still receive the healing, and that is how we take care of seven generations.[37]

This past August I was receiving chiropractic care for injuries received in a car wreck the month before. No matter what the doctor did, my shoulders and upper back would not release their hard, tight tension. I decided to explore and use symbolic sight to figure out what was going on with my body besides the car wreck. Symbolic sight means looking at life events in terms of universal archetypal patterns; it gives you a new view of yourself and others. Universal archetypes are typical, eternal, repeated motifs and behaviors manifested instinctually through the unconscious of a species. The Great Mother is one archetype that crosses all species. The ageless female or symbols such as Mother Bear, Mother Earth, Kuan Yin, and Virgin Mary are part of the Great Mother archetype. Dr. Jung elevated the concept of universal archetypes in his collective unconscious theory. He said, "… the archetypes impress, influence, and fascinate us…. They are part of the inherited structure of the psyche, which manifest spontaneously anywhere and anytime."[38]

I started by focusing on my subtle body and its main chakras (life or energy centers). The idea of a subtle body started with the Eastern or Hindu traditions of energy centers and fields. The subtle body interpenetrates our physical body. The auras, chakras, meridians, and nadis are part of this energy field or matrix. The subtle body is composed of the energetic field that surrounds each of us. This field extends as far out as your arms can reach and the full length of your physical body. When you are in a crowded elevator, bus, or when someone gets "in your face," that uncomfortable feeling and the need to move happens because someone has crossed into your subtle body boundary. The subtle body is an energetic blueprint for your SEMP health.

Most Eastern traditions teach about the subtle body and its chakras. The word *chakra* means "wheel," and like wheels, the chakras spin—how fast or slow depends on the energy system of the person. The chakras serve as the connecting points for our physical body and subtle body. Diseases usually appear in the subtle body as imbalances before manifesting as an illness in our physical body.

What does this have to do with wombology? Chakras regulate the flow of life energy in the physical body, and all of this life flow begins in the dark waters of your mother's womb. There are seven basic chakras, which correspond to certain physical systems, organs, and glands. When a part of your body speaks for your mind, there is a corresponding chakra, or voice. There is also a network of interconnecting energy channels called meridians (more on those later). The subtle body uses these meridians to deliver messages to us. Most of the time I use Caroline Myss's brief summary of the spiritual life lessons represented by the seven chakras to explore the energy system.

- First chakra: lessons related to the material world
- Second chakra: lessons related to sexuality, work, and physical desire

- Third chakra: lessons related to the ego, personality, and self-esteem

- Fourth chakra: lessons related to love, forgiveness, and compassion

- Fifth chakra: lessons related to will and self-expression

- Sixth chakra: lessons related to mind, intuition, insight, and wisdom

- Seventh chakra: lessons related to spirituality

Myss says, "The congruencies among major spiritual traditions underscore the universal human experience of the connection between the spirit and the body, illness and healing."[39]

Now do you see why the subtle body and chakras relate to wombology? By focusing on my chakras, deep breathing, and body movement, I realigned my chakras and moved on to work on the specific points on my body that were still holding tension.

The book, *Your Body Speaks Your Mind*, by Debbie Shapiro, contains a structural body-mind figure. I used it to explore how my body was speaking my mind. I colored in the areas that were filled with tension. Shapiro separates the body into three centers: from the neck up is the control center, from the neck to the waist is the doing center, and from the waist down is the moving center.[40] My tension involved the doing center, my shoulders and upper back. Symbolically, the shoulders are where we carry our responsibility; we carry other people's problems (OPP) or burdens. I call it cosigning for other people's problems.

According to Shapiro, my tense shoulders meant I was carrying too many burdens, cosigning for too many other people. She says the back represents the unconscious because it is where we dump issues or feelings that we don't want to deal with. Issues of survival are also connected to the back. The responsibility of being the "backbone" of the family is transferred through the back as well. So I realized that, symbolically, I was carrying the burdens of seven generations, and their pain and mine were lodged in my shoulders and upper back as well as in my cells. The horrors of slavery are part of my generational pain too.

After recognizing what was going on, I found a quiet space and place to meditate and pray to the souls of my seven generations. I asked to be released from all the pain that was lodged within my muscles. For the next three days I spent an hour to meditate with soft music while focusing on calling my energy and spirit back from my seven's zomai, or soulful cave. On the third day I got relief; my shoulders and back felt energized and lighter. Were the cell memories of seven generations released? I would like to think so. The next time I went to the chiropractor, he was amazed that my muscles and nerves had finally relaxed. Something within me was given permission to relax and play. My inner child could finally be responsible for just her stuff and yet allow me to still be accountable to all seven generations.

Now it's time for my personal wombology story. While I was jostling around in my grandmother's daughter's womb, she was already tending to her other three children, born just one year apart from each other. There are two years' difference between my next sibling and me. I am Mom's baby. Mom married at a very young age. She was fourteen years old when she became pregnant with my sister, Linda, and fifteen years old when she gave birth to her. This happened back in the 1950s, when stigma was still attached to getting pregnant before marriage, especially in a country town in Oklahoma. Mom's pregnancy fostered constant feelings of guilt, shame, depression, and embarrassment, and that is some of what Linda received in the womb, along with love.

My sister has often battled clinical depression, feelings of guilt and shame without knowing why. By the time Mom had me, she was five years into the marriage and in a happier emotional state, so I came into the world with happy, confident, shame-free emotional states. I have not struggled with clinical depression or guilt; of course, it helps being the baby of the family too.

One day Mom and Linda were talking when my sister said, "I often have to deal with shame, guilt, and depression and don't know why. It's like I'm ashamed I was born or something."

"Linda, maybe those aren't your feelings but mine. You just described how I felt most of the time when I was pregnant with you. I am so sorry for having burdened you with all that."

"Why did I sometimes feel as if I was in the way?"

"Your daddy was trying to get into the professional baseball league when I got pregnant, and he had to give up that dream to take care of you and me. Maybe you picked up on that."

Last fall during one of my visits back home Mom, Linda, and I were sitting around having one of our many deep conversations when Mom said, "Let me apologize to both of you for any harm I did to either one of you while you were in the womb or while you were growing up." Mom's countenance and voice was like that of a fourteen-year-old girl. It was like we were all experiencing a peek at her inner child's world. My insight into wombology has helped us release some of the past.

The next two pages contain drawings of what carrying the needs, responsibilities, and accountabilities of seven generations feels like for me. On the pages after that I share pictures of my seven generations. On the page where there are seven women, the one of the little child is actually my daughter as a toddler; that picture of her represents one of my generations.

The picture of the lady with the scarf on her head is a picture of someone I don't know personally, but she represents my great-great-grandmother Charity.

The story behind the lady who represents Charity started back in 1988. I was working in a retail store in Pueblo, Colorado, helping a man decide which cologne he wanted to buy, when we started discussing his latest travels to Africa. He shared a large stack of pictures he had just developed. He showed me his favorites and told me the stories behind them. We finished the sale and he was off to his next adventure. About one hour later I noticed that he accidentally left one picture with me, and I have never been able to throw it away. When I was working on my seven-generation picture, this picture, which I had not seen in years, literally fell off a bookshelf (synchronicity). I looked at it with new eyes because the lady has an uncanny resemblance to Great-Grandma Annie.

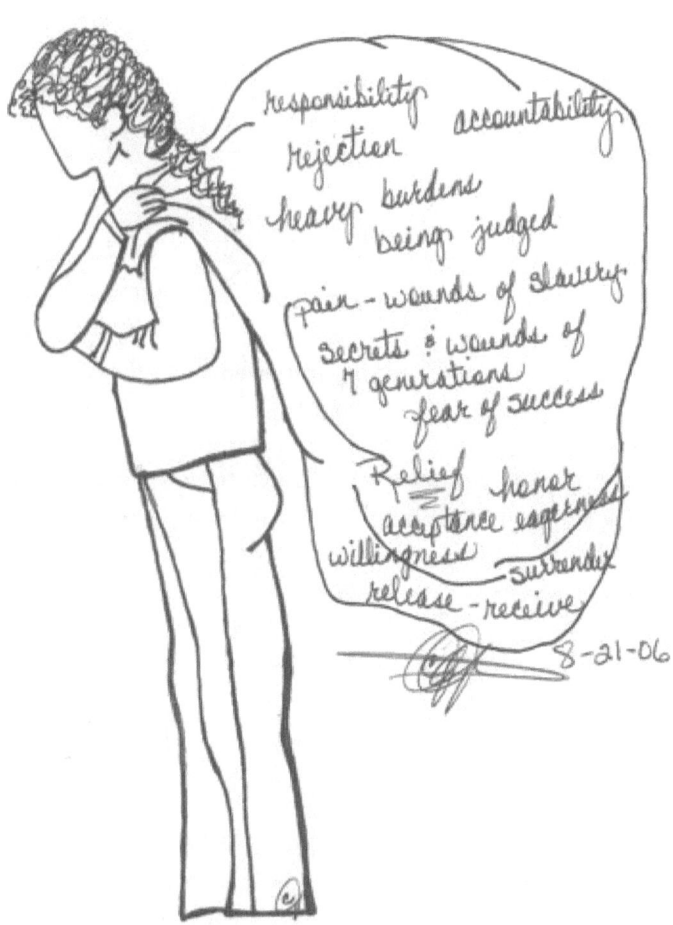

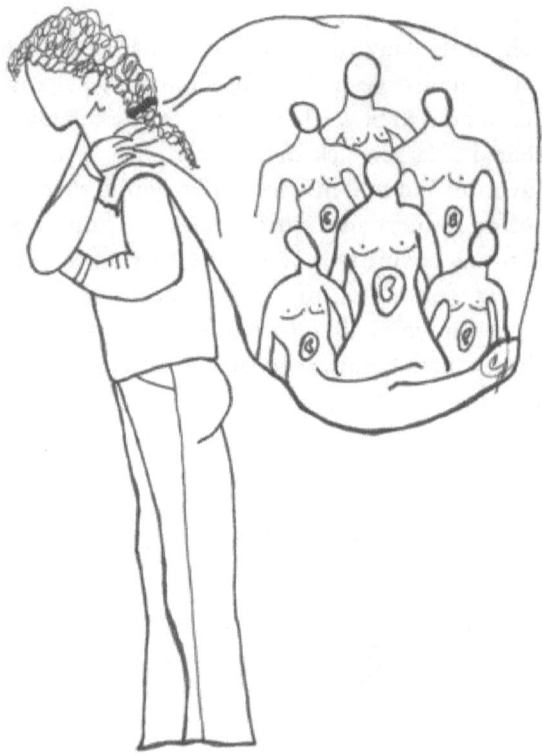

Carrying my seven

Are you aware that you carry seven generations of family? If not on your back, they are some where within your mind, body, or spirit.

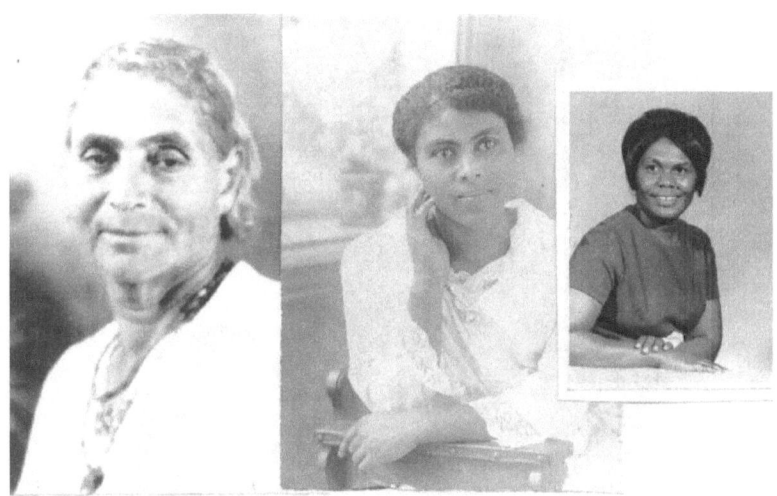

Mom Geraldine
Grandma Nellie
Great Grandma Annie

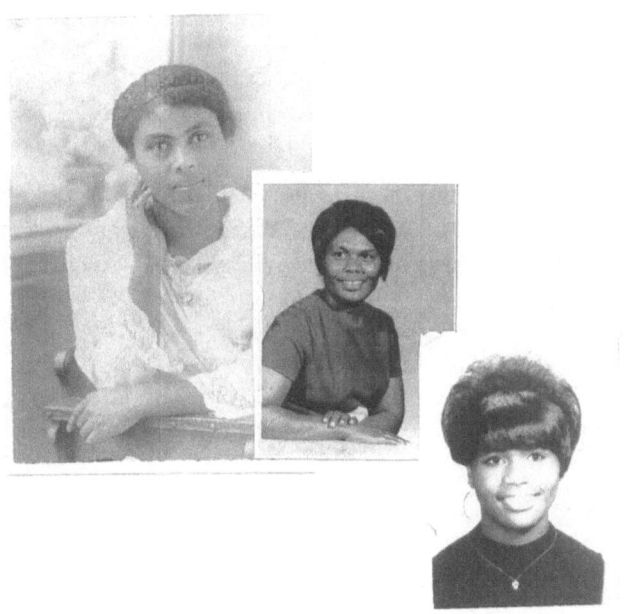

A pictorial motherhood genogram (Nellie, Geraldine, and C J).

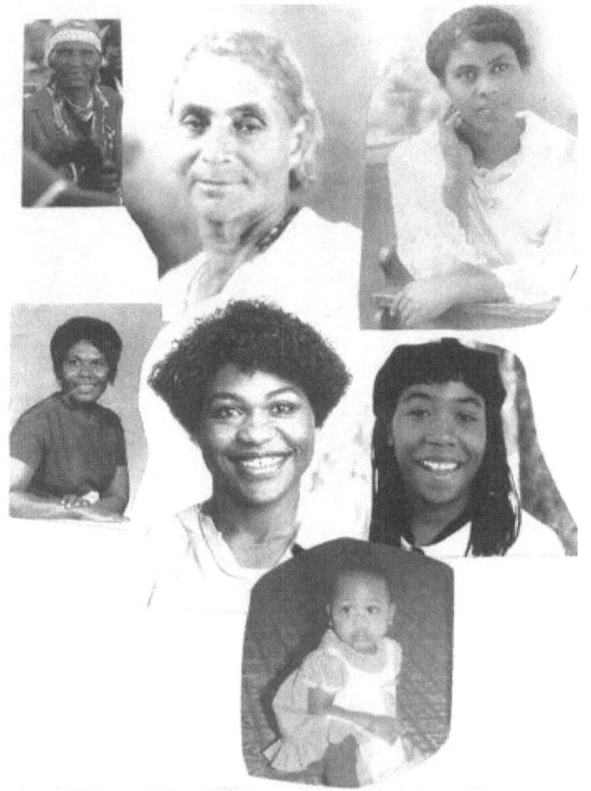

A visual representation of my "seven": A picture of an unknown African woman with family resemblance to represent Great-Grandma Charity, along with Annie, Nellie, Geraldine, C J, Chakira, and a baby picture of Chakira to represent the seventh.

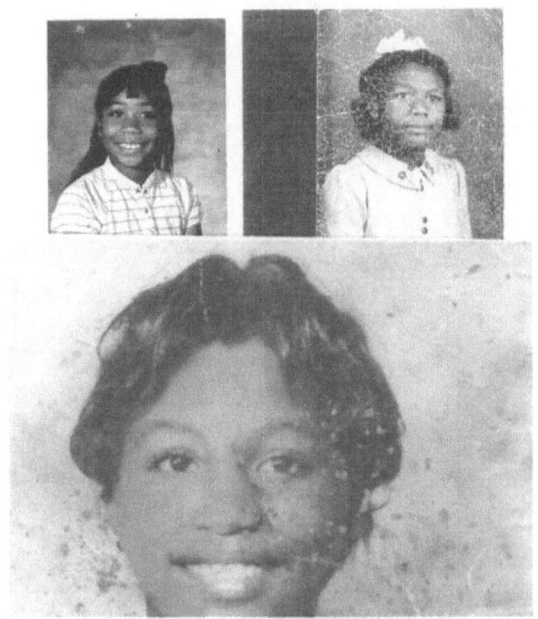

Chakira, Geraldine, and C J all at about age nine.

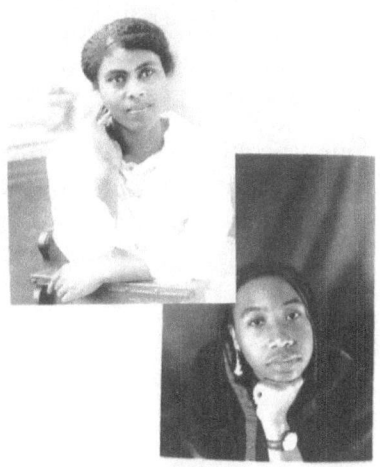

Shannon Richter©
Nellie (birth date March 11, 1891) and Chakira (birth date March 10, 1978).

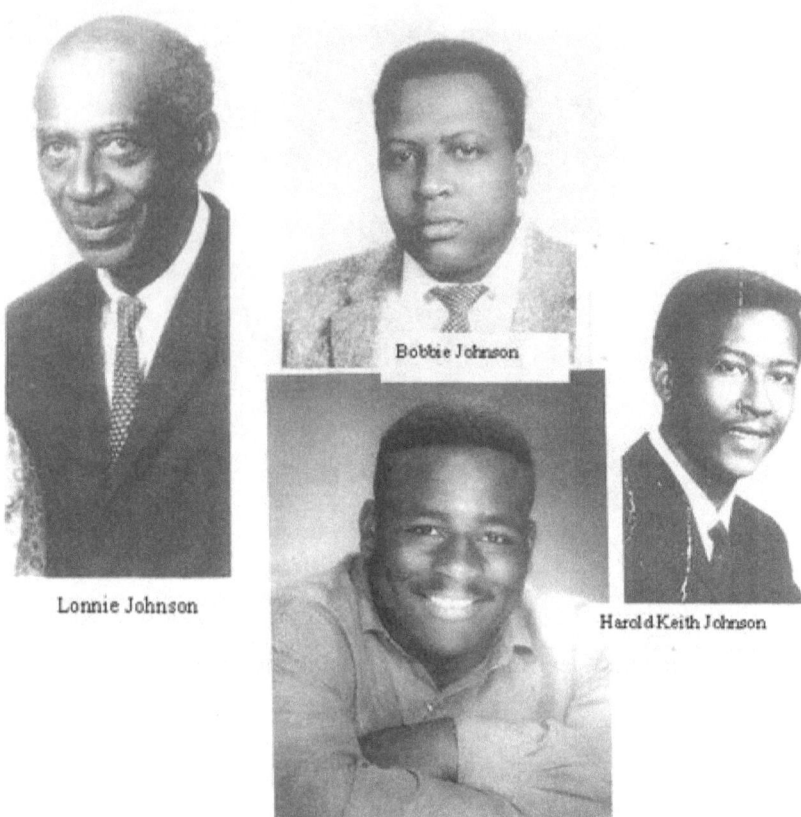

My husband and his four generations of Johnsons: his grandfather Lonnie, father Bob, himself, Harold Keith, and our son, Roddrick.

6

Warning: Inner Child at Play

✦

Whether you believe in the inner child concept or not, the inner child lives within all of us. It affects our daily life. The inner child is the child we once were, the little one who attempted to go through the development stages of Erikson and Bradshaw. This inner child continues to exist in our adult life and reflects our emotional health at any given moment. Our wounded inner child is a reflection, or a mirror image, of our disowned emotions left over from childhood. Our healthy inner child is a reflection of our claimed nurtured emotions.

If you want to witness the wounded inner child at work in others, tune into my favorite Friday night television series, TLC's *What Not to Wear*. On this show two fashion experts, Stacy London and Clinton Kelly, do a fashion intervention on a participant who was selected by a friend or family member and has agreed to be on the show. You will watch a person go from fashion-less to fashion-wise, from no confidence to self-confident, from no esteem to high self-esteem. Clinton and Stacy help people recognize that what they wear on the outside does not usually match who they are on the inside. I have noticed that eight out of ten times the person is stuck at a preteen age emotionally and therefore dresses inappropriate for her current age. The inner child throws a temper tantrum and becomes very resistant and protective of its symbolic childhood ponytail when the hair stylist, Nick Arrojo, tries to give the subject an adult haircut or style. It is a study of an inner child in action as he tries to calm the little one's fears and resistance to growing up.

Stacy and Clinton may not be aware of this, but they are helping their participants heal their inner child. I love watching the show as the participant transforms from wounded inner child to a self-confident adult, starting with the clothes they wear, letting go of the symbolic ponytail, and ending with the new way they perceive themselves during and after the transformation.

The world of the inner child begins in the womb. Whether that world is nurtured or neglected throughout childhood depends on so many things. People who have been rejected in the womb and again in childhood tend to be easily hurt, bitter, or hostile growing up, and it continues until they become this hurt, bitter, or hostile adult who cannot figure out what went wrong nor when. Too often an unwanted pregnancy leads to an emotionally disowned, abandoned child who becomes an adult with the same issues.

Often during individual therapy sessions I sense a change of energy in the room, usually indicated by the body language or demeanor of the client. That is when I ask, "Who just entered the room with us?"

The client usually asks, "What do you mean by that?"

I respond, "I mean all of a sudden it feels like someone who hurt you is in your head, and if that person is in your head, he or she is in this room with us right now."

Usually with a wide mouth and a strange peek at me, the client will admit who she was thinking about or a past situation that came to mind. Nine times out of ten it is something that happened during their childhood.

Your current age does not matter when you do inner child work, because if you have not liberated, explored, or acknowledged your inner child, it is still throwing temper tantrums and directing your life. The tantrums play out as addictions, fetishes, perfectionism, attachment disorders, and other forms of emotional chaos. Suppressing the inner child affects our daily life whether we are eighteen years old or eighty years old. Remember my aunt and her spankings?

My sister and I present Inner Healing Journey workshops in which inner child work is an intricate part. During workshops it is amazing to watch the adult participant's inner child symbolically enter the room. This usually happens when we are playing with crayons and using our non-dominant hand. At one of these we had an eighty-year-old woman who was holding on tightly to her eight year old inner child's pain of being emotionally and verbally mistreated by her father. Because of one phrase he uttered, she felt unloved and that she did not belong to her family of origin. Tears rolled down her cheeks as she said, "I often wonder if there is someone out there who can love me for me."

Now mind you, she had a mother and siblings who showed her love, but she chose to stay focused on her father's injurious words. A group hug and coloring with crayons while using her non-dominant hand helped her close a seventy-two-year-old open wound. She held this wound in secrecy and shame because she believed this was her own private pain and her cross to bear.

Can you remember being eight years old? Now imagine being treated like the dirty dishrag, a part of the family because of your functionality, not because you are loved. That was this woman's perception, and remember, your perception becomes your reality.

Bradshaw discusses the child's sense of his own value and dignity being precarious and that it needs to be mirrored and echoed from a nurturing caregiver. If the child does not get that reflection, he will lose the sense of being special and unique. That sounds a lot like my term *eye-love* and the Japanese *amae*. Bradshaw also states, "A child must first be loved before he can love."[41] So how can you love yourself or anyone else if you were not loved as a child?

On the subject of spiritual wounds Bradshaw says, "Every child needs desperately to know that (A) his parents are healthy and able to take care of him and (B) that he matters to his parents. Mattering means that the child's specialness is reflected in the eyes of his parents or other significant caretakers. Mattering is also indicated by the amount of time they spend with him. Children know intuitively that people give time to what they love. Parents shame their children by not having time for them."[42] If the reflection (mirror neuron) is unhealthy, how can you expect to be completely healthy?

W. Hugh Missildine, M.D., a psychiatrist and author of *Your Inner Child of the Past*, said, "Just as trees are shaped by the soil in which they grow, by the sun, the winds, and the rain, so did the climate created by your parents' attitudes influence your emotional development and outlook."[43] I consider the womb and its constant state the soil that shapes the unborn child. Doctor Jung said, "Nothing has a stronger influence psychologically on their environment and especially on their children than the unlived life of the parent."[44] That statement is one of the reasons I use the motherhood genogram to explore the generational "stuff" of the client. My experience is that too many people in therapy are really dealing with their parents' or grandparents' unresolved issues. Often people are dealing with generations of pain unknowingly passed on from one generation to another.

If your caretakers or parents were predictable, you learn to trust your needs will be met and the outside world is a warm place waiting to help you. If your caretakers or parents were unpredictable and you did not get your needs met, you learn to not trust and the outside world is a frightening place waiting to hurt you. Unfulfilled needs predispose you to develop maladjustments and to accept or give abusive behavior. That is not to say every person who did not get his needs met will react to his world with disorders, maladjusted behaviors, or abuse. But research shows that most people who are challenged with emotional dis-ease or use abuse to control and communicate are wounded people with unmet needs from their childhood. I know that only wounded people try to injure others.

The inner child's favorite dance is the FOOLISH ghost dance. Many times the child is reacting to the internal conflict of, "I was wounded the most by those people I loved the most." It is difficult to resolve that the people or person you trusted the most, loved the most, and needed the most as a child betrayed you and left you exposed when they should have covered you and protected you with love. I watch adults wrestling with the mind-set and attitudes of their parents even when their parents are no longer a part of their daily life. Clients continue to apply family untruths to themselves as if they were still children. Childhood brainwashing or family untruths get reinforced through repetition for the first eighteen years of life, and many people spend the next twenty to forty years trying to either live up to or dismiss the lies. Why? The untruths get recorded in our LTM and encoded at a cellular level within our bodies. Too many adults have built their world on a Jell-O-like foundation from childhood; this shaky foundation creates problems in almost every area of adult life.

Injurious parents are my number one form of job security; bullying teachers come in second. So many of my clients had teachers who bullied them during elementary school. When Cleo, a forty-year-old woman, first came to me, her main issue was with her daughter, you know that special mother-daughter relationship. As therapy progressed, we learned that a big part of her trying to prove to her own daughter that she was not stupid started with her third grade teacher. Cleo was still trying to prove to that teacher, Mrs. Williams, that she was not dumb or stupid and that Mrs. Williams was wrong for making her feel that way in front of the whole classroom. It also did not help the situation that Cleo was an unwanted pregnancy. Her mother doted on Cleo's younger sister. And so the pain goes on and on.

Jon, the adopted client discussed in chapter one, had a similar experience, but the teacher convinced both his parents that he belonged in the "slooow classes," so he would stop disrupting the "normal" kids. Forty years ago teachers had a lot of power, and most parents believed that teachers were so smart and knew exactly what was best for their children. Wrong again. Jung also said, "An understanding heart is everything in a teacher and cannot be esteemed highly enough. One looks back with appreciation to the brilliant teachers but with gratitude to those who touched our human feelings. The curriculum is so much necessary raw material, but warmth is the vital element for the growing plant and for the soul of the child."[45] I agree. I have many teachers I hold dear, but especially my second grade teacher, Mrs. Haigler, who told me often, "Carol, you are so smart you can be anything you want to be. I really believe that." Mind you, this was back in the 1960s, during the Civil Rights era. I want to be clear that adults other than parents can help or hurt a child for a lifetime.

If you are ready to reclaim your inner child beyond what we do in this book, a great place to start is with highly acclaimed author and inner child expert Lucia Capacchione's, *Recovery of Your Inner Child* and John Bradshaw's *Homecoming: Reclaiming and Championing Your Inner Child.* Be sure to check out my suggested reading list in the back of the book; those resources will help you with this healing journey. Dr. Capacchione shows us how to recover our inner child with exercises in her book. My favorite one is using the non-dominant hand. It is okay to be skeptical about using this technique, but stay open-minded—it really works. I have discovered many of my own internal, unwrapped gifts and processed anger issues by using my non-dominant hand.

If as a child you got your basic nurturing needs met, you would be a completely different person today. But since you did not, let's deal with it now. Find the energy to love yourself enough to let go of the hurtful past. Your inner child's pleas are, "Take care of me, play with me, listen to me, and believe in me." Find a safe, comfortable, quiet, space and invite your inner child to join you in a more healthy way. To become whole on SEMP levels, you will want to find out what you can do now to help integrate the curiosity, creativity, intuitiveness, and spontaneity of your inner child with the adult's responsibility, accountability, and reliability. This is imperative; personal and spiritual growth involves healing your inner child.

It sounds strange coming from me, the right-brained person, but in order to reclaim your own power it is best to use both hemispheres of the brain. Using both your dominant and non-dominant hands during an exercise allows both sides to get into the mix. Try one of these self-exploration exercises: Use your non-dominant hand to write or draw something that represents your story. Or, draw two pictures— one of you as a happy child and one as a sad child. Next, sit quietly for a few minutes while contemplating your story. After reflecting on your story, write it out with your non-dominant hand. And remember, if you nurture the hole in your heart, it will grow. If you nurture your whole heart, it will grow. Choose what will grow and direct your day.

Children have a different set of priorities than we do as adults, and our agenda is different as well. During this get-acquainted stage, do not make promises to your inner child that you have no intention of keeping. The key is to nurture and do no more harm. You have suffered long enough.

Now let's explore more about the younger you. Get your journal or a couple of sheets of paper and write the following questions. Or chose one from each set that is most meaningful to you and work with it. Use your dominant hand to write the question and your non-dominant hand to answer the question. Go with it until the thought plays itself out or nothing else comes to mind. Here are some questions I came up with for you to try. If they do not resonant with you, make up your own or find someone who specializes in inner child work to help you.

Questions
As a child, were you most often ... ?

1. Fearful
2. Social
3. Antisocial
4. Lonely
5. Moody
6. Sensitive
7. Needy
8. Difficult
9. Happy

What kind of attitudes did your parents or other caretakers have toward you as a child?

1. Overindulgent
2. Punitive
3. Angry
4. Neglectful
5. Excessive
6. Overbearing
7. Demanding
8. Depressed
9. Jealous

What were you to your mother?

1. I was expected to save her marriage.
2. I was going to rescue her from loneliness.
3. I absorbed her pain.
4. I was her protection.
5. I was her anger, guilt, or shame.

"Okay, Dr. C J, now that I've opened up all this, what now?" you ask. Letting go of wombology or woundology is very difficult work, even when you are ready and willing. It does not always happen easily or quickly, but for some there can be instant release or letting go. Just for today, release what you can. Use your favorite and most effective way to let go of unneeded stuff, or you can use one of mine. I love symbolism and if you do, too, try what I call the balloon solution. Find a small balloon. As you blow it up, symbolically let your wounds from your wombology or childhood enter the balloon's womb. Hold it in your hands and caress or massage it as your release stuck emotions or memories. Let the air out of it slowly. As you do, proclaim your victory over your wounds, whether received in the womb or childhood. Or you can tie the balloon, take it outside, and let it float up and away into the atmosphere as your weary wounds ascend and disappear.

Use whatever will work for you to help you to release that heavy, controlling pain of the past. This will empower you again. If at anytime you feel uncomfortable before or while you are doing this exercise, stop. Take this opportunity to breathe out loud, and consider having someone with you as a safety net, before you go deeper into the discomfort. This resistance and discomfort is normal and a part of the inner healing journey. Releasing your wombology does not mean it will not return. As a matter of fact, it may return when certain triggers or other memories pop up, but its intensity, duration, and power lessens each time it returns.

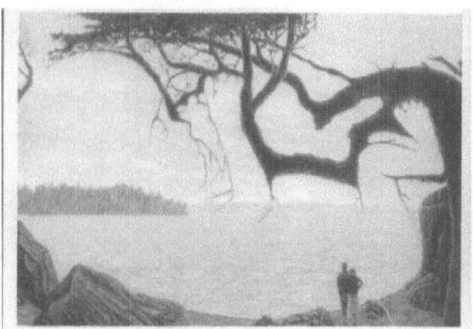

artist unknown

In this picture of a young couple enjoying the beautiful lakeside view, the tree and rocks seem to give them added privacy and protection. As you look softly at the whole scene, can you see the baby in the womb in this picture? If not, pull the page away from you a little more and focus softly on the shape of the tree branches.

Once you can see the baby, you cannot ignore it, which reminds you,

"Once awake, don't go back to sleep."

7

Growing Beyond the PAST

✦

Are you excited yet? I hope so. This is one of the most important chapters in the whole book, because if you have read this far you are ready to do something different. You are eager to finally give your old voices new choices, to own what is yours, and let go of what is not. Are you ready to put away stifling things (PAST)? You will explore, study, and reframe your life's story. If you allow your life's events to become a story, you can detach enough to view yourself through different eyes. Whose eyes? Maybe for the first time you will use your lens without your grandmother's daughter's blinders. Let's explore and *see* (pun intended) who or what pops up.

The best way to move beyond your pain is to let go of shame and blame. Let's go back to the fetus for a minute. The human heart develops in the fetus before the thinking brain, which means we feel things before we have the ability to use cognitive skills to think about things. Your heart will allow you to move forward, while your brain can keep you stuck in the past. In order to move on you will need to use both your heart's intelligence and your brain's intelligence. Stop living just in your head and get into real life instead.

The heart is constantly communicating with every cell in your body. That communication is what causes a gut reaction to someone or something. This same communication causes the butterflies in your stomach when you are with someone special. Think about this: when you get hurt, it is the heart that aches, not the brain. The ancient Egyptians had it right when they believed the heart was the source of wisdom, emotions, memory, and the seat of the soul, not the brain. Dr. Pearsall's book *The Heart's Code*, which I mentioned in chapter one, supports the Egyptians' theory.

Alignment of the mind, body, and spirit is the pathway to healing with permanence. So read the previous paragraph one more time to make sure you understand how important listening to your body can be. Let's get started. We will use the SMART (specific, measurable, achievable, related to goal, and time-limited) steps to work through recovering from past wounds.

If you work through these seven stages successfully, they will help you move beyond your injurious wombology.

The Seven Stages of Growth and Recovery

1. Awareness
2. Investigation
3. Discomfort
4. Reflection
5. Preparation
6. Action
7. Release

- *Awareness.* Everyone on this planet has had a womb experience, even your mother, father, grandmothers, and grandfathers. Watch *In the Womb*, a DVD produced by National Geographic. It will raise your awareness of how much a fetus can learn and retain while in the womb, and it will make you curious about your womb-time. Ask your mom or grandmother what they know about their womb-time.

- *Investigation.* Ask family members or friends what they know about the times before your conception, as well as your womb-time. Look through historical time line books to get a feel for the climate of the time at least one year before your conception and the time during your gestation period.

- *Discomfort.* You are not sure why, but you do not feel whole or healthy. There is this recurring theme or nagging presence in your life that will not go away. You no longer are comfortable with all the rational lies you have been telling yourself to make the world okay. You want to do something different, but you are not sure what that could be. Besides, all this exploration takes you outside of your comfort zone. Discomfort is part of the process; do not resist it.

- *Reflection.* "I know, I know," you say. You know what to do (or not to do), but you do not do it. Now is the time to reflect on what is preventing you from being who you want to be. What part have you played wittingly or unwittingly with the results in your life right now? Whom do you need to ask for forgiveness? Who have you put into therapy? Who would benefit the most from a healed you? The universe is waiting on you to be of service not only to your seven generations, but to others as well.

- *Preparation.* You have had your "aha" moment, gathered womb-time information, read most of this book, and have talked with those people who can help you move forward. You are preparing spiritually, emotionally, mentally, and physically for the change that is right around the corner. Light your favorite candle or incense to symbolize your journey's new beginning.

- *Action.* Get on your mark. Get set. Go. Work through the exercises on the following pages. Get out some paper and design the life of your dreams. Write down your vision of what your optimal life will be and let your heart's intelligence lead the way. Let go of attachment to a specific outcome. Everything you need to heal is with you right now.

- *Release.* Letting go is not easy, but when you find inner peace (serenity), the outer piece will fall into alignment. Let go of all those unmet childhood needs. Let go of all those expectations of your parent(s) loving you exactly the way you needed. Let go of childish things that no longer serve you. Let go of negative beliefs. Let go of self-criticism and self-sabotage. It is your time and turn.

No one else can do this work for you, but I can help lead the way as you move through your stuff. That's right—this time it is all about you and your past! Let's get started.

What should you expect? What changes will happen? Expect to be able to let go of blaming others for your place in life. You will learn how to reframe some of the life-changing events in your life. Expect that as you get healthy, so will your parenting skills. Expect to stop living in your head (memories), which keeps parts of you dead. Expect self-acceptance, self-worth to improve, and self-esteem to climb. And last but not least, expect to find forgiveness for the wounded people who have injured you, including yourself. The hardest thing is to forgive yourself for something you could have done differently.

Once you realize that your wombology is not a part of your DNA, that it is not your whole story and it can be changed, you can become the healthy generation. Once you have examined your story, your truth, you cannot just pick yourself up, act as if nothing happened, and go back to your old ways of being or doing. You have just cleared your psyche. What purpose would be served for you to go backwards? Why continue to harm yourself with your past once you are awake and aware of it on a conscious level? Self-knowledge takes the sting out of the old wounds. Socrates' quote, "An unexamined life is not worth living," fits this healing process.

After exploring and witnessing your wounds, investigate how these wounds continue to affect your daily life. Do not wallow in your anger, pain, or abandonment issues, even if you currently practice Bowenian emotional cutoffs (where you pretend a family member does not exist or where you simply choose to not engage with a family member). Allow your feelings to surface; when you deny them, they start controlling you and your inner child throws yet another tantrum. Just let the story of your feelings unfold and look at the story from a new percept.

Internal work can be confusing, scary, disheartening, disorienting, and sometimes downright pain-filled. On the other hand, it can be fun, insightful, directive, informative, and enlightening. This probably sounds chaotic, and it very well can be, but all of this chaos has a purpose and is part of the process. This is a journey only the courageous can take. My definition of *courageous* is knees shaking, stomach jumping, and scared witless for a quick second, but you do it anyway. To paraphrase Albert Einstein, every day we have to act as if everything in life is a miracle or as if nothing in life is a miracle. You are the miracle.

Okay, let's generate your genogram, like mine in chapter two. Remember, this is not about assigning blame or shame but about exploring from whence you came. Get a sheet of paper and make three two-prong loops or an elongated *u*. Put your father's name on the left side and mom's on the right, and make the same above that with your grandparents' names. Make one more above them with your great-grandparents' names, like the example below.

This genogram will make your pre-wombology history visual by gathering and using the gleaned information. Explore the relationships between the males and females before or during a pregnancy with the following helps.

- *Acknowledge* births, deaths, divorces, emotional cutoffs, constant emotional states, and unresolved grief at least one year before or during the same time frame.

- **Questions** to ponder: were there any domestic violence, incestuous relationships, addictions, depression, mental, or physical health issues that could affect your story? How does your genogram play out? Does it illuminate new information or put old information in a new light?

- **Birth order** makes a difference. Remember my wombology and the difference between my sister, who is the oldest of four, and me, the youngest. According to the late psychoanalyst Alfred Adler, birth order can determine societal and familial expectations of you.[46] Sometimes those expectations can help you or hinder you in the process of healing.

One part of the process of inner healing is to acknowledge and appreciate the woman who brought you into the world for doing the best that she could at that time. Give thanks for your life, and as part of the healing, forgive and release anything you received from your mother that has been less than helpful to you. Read the book *Forgive Your Parents, Heal Yourself: How Understanding Your Painful Family Legacy Can Transform Your Life*, by Dr. Barry Grosskopf. If you are ready, it has the power to transform your perception of your parents' lives and therefore yours. Grosskopf tells vivid stories of how children are imprinted with the outmoded and outdated responses and how absorbing emotions of parents or grandparents influence daily life. One of my favorite parts in this book is when Grosskopf discusses the scripture that I mentioned in chapter two, Jeremiah 31:29: "The fathers have eaten a sour grape, and the children's teeth are set on edge." That is the perfect description of wombology. Family secrets can keep a whole family sick and injure future generations.[47]

Too often future generations carry and respond to the unshed tears or unhealthy debris of past generational injuries. We have to find a way to stop passing on outdated and ineffective survival reactions, long-held resentments, and unresolved grief as generational baggage or unnamed pain. Forgiveness is the key to healing all seven generations.

Forgiveness is not for the person who injured you but for you. As long as you hold on to resentment, hate, and anger for someone who hurt you, you hold tightly on to someone who is still in control of different aspects of you. Sometimes you are afraid to let go because you don't know for sure what would happen if you did, so you hang on to anger-security. Emotionally or symbolically, you are still holding on to some part of the person who hurt you in the past. Hanging on to frozen resentment is like drinking ipecac and hoping the person across the room will vomit for you. It ain't gonna happen.

You have to make a conscious decision to let go and forgive for your own sake. Sometimes I wish I had a magic wand and a swift, easy solution to this emotionally charged paradox. But I do not. Letting go of old emotional debris is not easy, but it is worth it.

Forgiveness can happen when you least expect it and in an instant. I witnessed this often with clients and one day with Keith. When my husband was growing up, his father, Bob Johnson, did not show him love, validation, or nurturing. Keith was the outsider looking in as his father showed affection for nieces, nephews, and his "other" family. Keith felt that his father thought of him last, even though he was his father's firstborn. To make matters worse, Keith looked just like his father, which made it harder to accept his father's rejection of him. They never really got the chance to establish a loving father-son relationship. My children were adults before they saw their first picture of their grandfather, who had been deceased for more than twenty-five years. His name was not mentioned in our home without being sandwiched between some spicy curse words by Keith.

One day two years ago I asked Roddy, "If you could go back into time and talk to anyone, who would it be?" My mouth flew open and my eyes bugged when he said, "Bob Johnson."

"Why, Bob?" I asked without thinking.

"I would like to thank him for giving me the father I have today. Because Bob was such a s— a—, Dad decided he would be the opposite and be the best father he could be. And I would just like to thank Bob for it."

Later in the day when I shared this revelation with my husband, he looked at me through wide dewy eyes and said, "When you look at it like that, I guess it was not all bad."

That was an "aha" moment and a life-changing event for him. In that instant, his frozen anger, hurt, and hate were defrosted and he was able to start to forgive his father for being just a sperm donor. Keith's inner child was able to see his father in a new light and to reframe some of his childhood experiences with him

I thought about the scripture "and a little child shall lead them" (Isaiah 11:6). What a miracle! Keith and I had been married for thirty-three years, and I never expected him to be able to move beyond his childhood pain or to hear him say, "I can never love him, but I no longer hate him and want to beat him down." Our thirty-year-old child led his father to forgiveness and a new view. I guess there are days when even our wounds are sick and tired of being sick and tired and waiting to be released. If you can't let go of your injurious past, find a way at least to let it rest so that you can move forward.

If you are ready and willing to let go of your harmful wombology, start with, "I thank you and forgive you for making me who I am today. From this day forward I will be me, not us. I am letting the universe absorb what I no longer want or need to facilitate my alignment and continued personal growth." A core belief for me is that when Jesus asked his father to forgive them ("for they know not what they do," Luke 23:34), he was asking his father to forgive others and me for the mistakes yet to be made. He was not just talking about those people who were standing around his feet mocking him or those who crucified him all those years ago. He was also talking about me and others who came after him.

As a spiritual midwife, part of my duties is to help others recognize that in order to make a conscious new birth, we have to be awake and aware of the present moment. We have to take inventory of habits and beliefs that no longer serve our best interests and may be hindering our spiritual growth. In her book *Anatomy of the Spirit*, Caroline Myss states, " We are biological creations of Divine design. Once this truth becomes a part of your conscious mind, you can never again live an ordinary life."[48] I agree and believe that is why you need to know where you are right now SEMP.

Your motherhood genogram should have answered a lot of questions for you so that you can start to live your extraordinary, divine life, which includes working your purpose, mission, and a meaningful life for seven generations. So many people are in search of *purpose*; it is quite simply *service* to the universe. Our *mission* is to *grow spiritually*, and living a *meaningful* life means *sharing your gifts* with the universe. That is how you take care of your seven generations.

The next tool of recovery from your wombology helps you develop a sense of who your mother was before you became a part of her story, and it gives you a chance to symbolically and historically walk a mile in her shoes. This will help you view, acknowledge, and understand some of the experiences of the most influential person in your life with enough detachment and objectivity to "get it." As author Helen Exley said, "Whether you like it or not, your mother goes with you. Forever."[49]

You will become a life scene investigator (LSI). (Yes, the TV series *CSI: Crime Scene Investigation* influenced my choice of title.) You will study the evidence or story of one of the most meaningful persons in your life and let that story unfold enough to gather a clear understanding of many of the unknown chapters that went into your wombology. It is your way of calling your spirit and energy back into this moment and inside your internal boundaries, where you are more in control. I have included a worksheet in this chapter for you to use to call your spirit back. In the meantime, it is your turn to play the detective and find out what is waiting for you to acknowledge or claim.

Remember the picture of the fetus in the branches of the tree in the previous chapter? Once you see it, you cannot pretend that you do not.

Now it is time for you to see the infant in your family tree that may have been wounded in the womb. It is time for you to wake up and stay awake. In the wonderful book *The Magic of Forgiveness: Emotional Freedom and Transformation at Midlife,* author Tian Dayton wrote, "I am carrying something inside of me that is undermining my happiness and stealing my joy. I am sick and tired of holding onto this pain. No matter where it started or who it belongs to, it belongs to me now. It lives inside of me, disturbs my peace of mind and exacts a heavy price; and I am just as sick of my own self-recrimination, of holding something against myself, of hurting my own inner world because I can't let myself or someone who is living in my head and heart off the hook. I am blocked in some way that I don't fully understand, but I'm willing to take a leap of faith into my inner world to look for some answers. I'm slowly coming to the conclusion that whatever grudge or resentment or wound I'm carrying is costing me more than I want to pay. I am waking up, seeing things differently, and willing to take a deeper look."[50] What a relief to say that out loud and finally let it go! Stop waiting; exhale.

Now, let's take a deeper look by using the worksheets on the following pages. I designed these exercises to facilitate your journey, but not as a quick fix. Working through these sheets takes time, energy, and courage. You cannot bypass it; you cannot rush it or hush it. I hope you use these tools as a graceful way to help find your place and space, to be yourself, and to become whole from the inside out. If you still feel scattered or fragmented, slow down long enough to go through this personal scavenger hunt and find the treasure within you. I know there are many people, even experts in the healing field, telling you, "Just get over it. Let the past be the past." Well, my friend, if that is all it took, everyone would be "over it" and healthy. I would have no reason to write this book, and you certainly would not be reading it. You cannot lie to yourself and heal yourself at the same time.

Sometimes we have a tendency to lie to ourselves or be in total denial about how others experience or respond to us. The Johari window is an excellent tool to determine how other people experience us. It gets its name from the first names of the two men who developed it in 1955, Joe Luft and Harry Ingram.[51] This tool will teach you about self-disclosure and feedback, both of which can help you understand how your interpersonal communications and relationships affect others or how they experience you.

If you and your mother drive each other crazy, that craziness could have started in the womb. Here is a tool that will help you stop the insanity of unhealthy conflict or the drain from one of you being an energy thug. You have been around people who are energy thugs, but they have no clue that they are draining you. The question to ask yourself is, "How often am I an energy thug?" We all are from time to time, but if that is your everyday mode of operating, you just might want to do something different.

How can you tell if you are an energy thug? If you notice people inhaling deeply as you walk toward them or if they inhale loudly during your conversations, you might be an energy thug. If people unconsciously but constantly cross their arms while listening to you, you just might fit the description. Energy thugs rarely listen to other people's stuff—they are mostly about themselves. Sometimes they will pause long enough to inhale and you think they are listening to you, but after they exhale the conversation goes right back to them. Does this sound like you at all?

This tool will help you and the people with whom you interact. The Johari window is divided into four quadrants or panes: public, blind, secret, and unconscious. Quadrant One (known to self and others) is the public self. Quadrant Two (unknown to self and known by others) is the blind self. Quadrant Three (known to self and unknown to others) is the secret self. Quadrant Four (unknown to self and to others) is the unconscious self.

The panes vary in size according to where you are at in your life when you use this assessment tool. Each quadrant's size can and will change over time. Remember, the purpose of the Johari window is to help you become more aware of how you come off to others and determine what aspect of yourself you need to work on. Quadrant Two, the blind self, is a key window to work on so you can witness what others do when interacting with you. If you have a taxing relationship with someone, this is a great tool to use.

Thorny relationships are often the result of the inner child acting out its unmet needs, which people are exposed to without your awareness. For example, if other people constantly tell you that you are hyper, that means that is how most people experience you. Remember the client from chapter three who said through clenched jaws that he was not angry? That is how most people experienced him. After you become aware of your blind spots, find a way to diminish them. This helps everyone involved with you—even strangers—to walk away with a positive experience of you instead of a negative one or the feeling of, "What just happened here?"

One of the best ways to heal your inner child or apply salve to wounds that are chronic and ancient is through bodywork. Bodywork includes acupuncture, acupressure, massage, physical therapy, and chiropractic care. I highly recommend that you find a trusted bodywork practitioner. There are a plethora of specific types of bodywork to use in conjunction with the healing process. The three I love to use while exploring, digging, and healing are Myofascial Release Treatment, acupressure, and emotional freedom technique (EFT). These specific techniques will facilitate your journey, and the retrieval of self will have a much more sense of permanence.

If you can find a physical therapist who is trained in John F. Barnes's Myofascial Release Treatment (MFT), you will thank your blessed stars every time you have a session. I had one session with one of his master physical therapists at his center, Therapy on the Rocks, while on a spiritual retreat in Sedona, Arizona, and if I could afford it I would go there every other month. Instead, I have found an MFT therapist within five miles of my home, and I seek her treatments often.

John Barnes's book *Healing Ancient Wounds: The Renegade's Wisdom* is a great starting point. Many of the ancient wounds are from wombology. I use this book as one of my reference books and have the pages all marked up with Post-it flags and highlighting. MFT is a mind-body therapeutic healing approach that is gentle, consistent, effective, and produces lasting results. This technique uses sustained pressure on the connective tissue, or fascia, that runs throughout the whole body in a three-dimensional web. Barnes says, "The inner journey is not just the most important journey; it is the *only* journey!"[52] It is a healing journey worth taking.

Both acupressure and acupuncture are great forms of bodywork to integrate into your healing journey. I have had both types applied to me and prefer acupressure. Acupuncture is not painful, but the sight of all those needles in my body played mind games with me. Try them both and decide which one works best for you.

If you cannot find a practitioner who provides acupressure and who understands the connection between bodywork and emotional healing, start by reading the book Acupressure *for Emotional Healing,* by Michael R. Gach and Beth Henning. This book teaches you how to locate vital points on the body and how to apply pressure to those points. Acupressure uses the same meridians of acupuncture, but your hands are the tools instead of needles. The authors say, "We highly recommend that you work with a psychotherapist as a complement to support the depth of your emotional healing as you practice the self-care techniques for common complaints."[53] This healing journey is one that only you can take, but you do not have to take it alone.

Last but not least, if possible, find a practitioner who is trained in Emotional Freedom Technique (EFT), I use the one developed by Gary Craig. Visit the EFT Web site (www.emofree.com) to find practitioners in your area. EFT uses gentle but firm tapping on the body in a specific order, called The Recipe. The tapping, certain phrases, and The Recipe allow emotional relief, which leads to emotional and physical healing. This method greatly reduces the time spent in traditional psychotherapy. EFT gets to the emotional and energetic causes of disease, not just the physical or mental symptoms. Craig promises, "A journey toward emotional freedom is not a mythical ride on a magic carpet that ends in illusion. It is a real ride destined to give you real results."[54]

I promised I would tell you what I do to improve my whole-braininess so as not to remain just right-brained. As part of my ongoing mental growth, I use two scientifically proven acoustic therapies. Dr. Jeffrey Thompson, owner of the Center for Neuroacoustic Research and international teacher of behavioral psychoacoustics, has created many music and sound series that promote healing, relaxation, and self-awareness. My two favorites are Healing Mind System and Brainwave Massage (for both sides of the brain). His sound medicine resonates with me on a soulful level.

I also use the Holosync Solution, a self-mastery tool that uses audio technology, soothing environmental sounds, and Autofonix—silent communication technology—to help the listener go into the different brain waves states for meditations. The states are deep alpha, theta, and delta. This program also helps with whole brain integration, which you now know I need. Bill Harris, CEO of Centerpointe Research Institute and the Holosync Solution and an author, also recommends using the SMART system I mentioned earlier.

To make lasting changes in the new you, use the SMART tools I have developed: the motherhood genogram, the call your spirit back (CYSB) technique, the good-bye letter, and the letter of recommendation to help you move beyond your wombology. The late Joseph Campbell, author and longtime protégé of Carl Jung, said, "We must be willing to get rid of the life we've planned, so as to have the life that is waiting for us."[55] I add to that, "When you let go of what you are, you make room for who you are."

Before you get started with the exercises in this book, if you suffer with Posttraumatic Stress Disorder (PTSD), please consult with your therapist or health practitioner before attempting these exercises. PTSD is a difficult challenge and usually requires some type of professional help. Most of my clients who have PTSD do very well by reading the book *I Can't Get Over It: A Handbook for Trauma Survivors*, by Dr. Aphrodite Matsakis, as we work through their trauma and doing bodywork.

The following worksheets will be your partners on this voyage to self-discovery, building self-esteem, and receiving self-acceptance. Let's go!

LSI (Life Scene Investigation)

Birth date: _____

Were there any remarkable events during your nine months of development in the womb (for instance, Oklahoma City bombing, a president's death while in office)? _____
_____
_____
_____

What world events took place on your birthday or within a week of your birth? _____
_____
_____
_____

What family events took place on your birthday or within a week of your birth (marriage, divorce, birth, death, etc.)? _____
_____
_____

Do you know your mom and/or dad's emotional state while she was pregnant with you (happy, sad, shameful, etc.)? _____
_____
_____

What original message did you receive as a child (mistake, wanted, good, not good enough, etc.)? _____
_____
_____

Did the original message become a core belief (FOOLISH ghost dance)? ___
_____
_____
_____
_____

What current behavior supports the FOOLISH ghost dance (low self-esteem, feeling unworthy, etc.)? _____

_____

_____

_____

Do you recognize any unearned pain that you cannot explain (anger, depression, shame, etc.)? _____

_____

_____

_____

What is the original pain? _____

_____

_____

_____

Who or what reinforces your core belief about this situation? _____

_____

_____

_____

What lessons do you still need to experience or work through concerning the original message or core belief?

_____

_____

_____

_____

What chaos do you continually create that reinforces your core belief?

_____

_____

_____

_____

Has there been a life-changing event or insight? _____

_____

_____

Are you willing and ready to change your core beliefs concerning certain situations? _____

_____
_____

Whom do you need to forgive or give thanks to for your release from the wombology cycle of victim thinking or repeating the same old mistakes? ___
_____
_____
_____

Now, what is your core belief around this pain? _____
_____
_____
_____

Write or draw your original message or pain below using your non-dominant hand. Read it out loud three times and then symbolically scratch it out, bury it, or white it out of your system:

CALL YOUR ENERGY AND SPIRIT BACK
A WOMBOLOGY RECOVERY WORKSHEET

Date: _____ Subject: (*)_____ Worksheet #____

1. *Awareness:* I am carrying someone else's pain: _____
I know this is not my stuff because_____
_____
_____.
I don't know if it's my grandmother's or my mother's, but I do know I will no
longer carry the _____
_____ that has become generational. Today I will _____
_____
_____.

2. *Boundaries*: I'm not sure where I start and
(*)_____ stops, but today I am willing to draw
the line and _____
_____.

3. *Accountability:* I realize that I am accountable for my life from this moment
forward. I also realize you gave me _____
__ without intending to harm me. I am taking 100 percent accountability for
me, not us but me. I've been stuck in _____
_____, but I am through with that.

4. *Beliefs:* I've worn your lens long enough. I am viewing my SEMP life
through different eyes. I want to discover _____
_____.
I believe it is time for _____
_____
_____.

5. *Forgiveness:* (*)_____ is not about you; it is about me
moving on.
I forgive me for _____
_____
_____
_____
_____.

I forgive you for _____
_____
_____
_____
_____.

6. *Reframing:* I understand that your intent may have been different, but I can now find the gift in the pain of _____
_____. I can reframe what I received in the womb and not carry it to my tomb. Your fears have taught me to _____.
Your depression gave me _____.
Your anger showed me _____
_____.

7. *Action:* I am ready and willing to _____
_____ so that I can move beyond the wombology. I am calling my spirit back from our _____
_____. I no longer want to be a part of the energy drain on either of our souls'. I will _____
_____.

8. *Practice:* If my *soul* wrote a book about myself, what would the title be?
_____
_____

I will invite my soul into my daily life by _____
_____
_____
_____.

9. *Change:* This is how I can create my optimal life: _____
_____
_____
_____
_____

This is how I can move beyond what I no longer need: _____
_____
_____
_____

This is how I can create a better relationship with (*): _____
_____

Make no mistake about it: this process works whether your mother is still earthbound or has already crossed over to the other side. Only the body dies. Our soul/spirit is eternal and can still receive.

"Without freedom from the past, there is not freedom at all, because the mind is never new, fresh, innocent." —Krishnamurti, spiritual teacher

WRITE A GOOD-BYE LETTER

This letter has five essential levels; feel free to change it to fit your needs. The lead-in phrases below are just examples; write what works for your situation. Be sure to work through all five points. This is to remain an unsent letter. It is a symbolic release.

1. Anger and blame
   I'm so mad at you because ...
   I'm tired of you ...
   You owe me ...

2. Hurt and sadness
   I feel hurt whenever you ...
   I am disappointed because ...
   I feel sad because ...

3. Fear and insecurity
   I'm afraid of ...
   I feel scared when you ...
   I wish you would ...

4. Guilt and accountability
   I'm sorry that ...
   I didn't mean to ...
   I am guilty of ... and you are guilty of ...

5. Forgiveness and understanding
   I forgive me for ...
   I forgive you for ...
   Thank you for ...

Here is an example of one of the levels in a good-bye letter. This type of symbolic letter will help you release what is still hindering you.

Dear Mom,
I am so angry with you for allowing me to carry your unnamed pain. I am mad at you because I've mistreated you, others, and myself using your anger. I am tired of carrying your anger, shhhame, and guilt ....

Now that you have started on the road to freedom from your past and you have reframed your wombology story, I want you to write a character letter of recommendation for the new you. Then use this letter as your daily affirmation to the authentic you. This is a heart-to-soul communication. It is time to stop asking God to explain his "whys" and simply ask, "What does this mean to me? Is this a lesson, warning, or gift?"

A traditional letter of recommendation is designed to validate, support, and present a person you know and care about. Like all other letters, it has a beginning, middle, and end. The beginning has one paragraph of two or three sentences. The middle has one or two paragraphs with three or more sentences. The end has one paragraph with no more than two sentences. In this letter you will present your strong points and positive attributes.

Here are some positive attributes people often use in reference letters:

- Insightful, well rounded, well grounded, empathetic
- Trustworthy, credible, reliable
- Creative, detail-oriented, open-minded
- Responsible, intelligent, organized, patient
- Easy to get along with, team player, leader
- Ambitious, enthusiastic, energized
- Generous, fair, problem solver
- Attentive, good listener, levelheaded

Here is a sample letter I wrote about myself.

LETTER OF RECOMMENDATION SAMPLE

Salutation: To Whom It May Concern:

Beginning: I am honored to present and recommend C J Johnson. She is a wild and bodacious woman who lives passionately and zestfully. As a field hand for the universe, she is constantly doing service for others and shining her light on their darkness.

Middle: I have known C J for fifty-three years, and she has always been full of life, creative, energized, insightful, and well-grounded. She is ready to start a new phase of the rest of her life, and I believe she will achieve whatever she is reaching for because she is courageous enough to step out of the box.

Ending: I am proud to recommend C J for this opportunity to heal the wounded, weary souls and spirits that she encounters. She is an asset to our global community.

Humbly I am,
C J Johnson, PsyD

Whew! That was easier than I expected. Try it and see what you come up with for yourself. You will feel good about all your hard emotional work. If you do not find relief after all of this work, I'm through with you ... just kidding! Use your newfound LSI skills and keep digging for the evidence that there is a beautiful, unwrapped gift inside of you. If you need more professional help, seek it out. Please don't be the proverbial learner or seeker who never applies the new awareness into your daily life.

It is time for us to stop being afraid of life and stop our passive participation in life. Here is my favorite quote about fear by Marianne Williamson, which helps me step outside of my fears and comfort zone at the same time.

> Our deepest fear is not that we are inadequate. Our deepest fear is that we are powerful beyond measure. It is our light, not our darkness that most frightens us. We ask ourselves, who am I to be brilliant, gorgeous, talented, fabulous? Actually, who are you not to be? You are a child of God. Your playing small does not serve the world. There is nothing enlightened about shrinking so that other people won't feel insecure around you. We are all meant to shine, as children do. We were born to make manifest the glory of God that is within us. It's not just in some of us; it's in everyone. And as we let our own light shine, we unconsciously give other people permission to do the same. As we are liberated from our own fear, our presence automatically liberates others.[56]

Too often life gets in the way of living, and there will always be something you can use as an excuse to put off living fully, something that keeps your fears alive, and something that makes you think you are not worthy. But *now* is your time and turn.

Now is the time for you to stop waiting for:

• Your prince / soul mate

• Mother / father's love

• Your bliss

- A good night's sleep
- Energy to live your life
- Your ship to come in
- Your house to feel like your home
- Your adult children to grow up
- The right time to exhale

Many of my clients tell me, "C J, I want to be just like you when I grow up." My response is, the universe does not need another C J. What it needs is a healthy you. The universe is waiting for you to get it together. When you are healed, willing, and ready, you can bring your uniqueness to the round table of life and support someone else's spiritual growth and wombology recovery. Have a seat and a cup of comfort as you reflect on who you are truly meant to be. Hold on to those memories that empower you and encourage you to continue to move forward. Your health is your greatest wealth, and that health includes spiritual, emotional, mental, and physical.

Now is the time for you to go on a retreat, whether that retreat is for five minutes, one hour, one day, a weekend, or five days. You deserve time without someone asking, "What's wrong with you?" My portable retreat bag is one of those see-through, satin drawstring bags you can buy at your local craft store. In it I keep those things that allow me to breathe deeply and retreat long enough to regroup, revitalize, and recognize that I either created this chaos or it is not about me. My bag always contains a journal, four or five different colored gel pens, a badge that declares my inner child is at play, music, and, of course, the Serenity Prayer. I first started using this prayer when I worked on the CDU in Colorado. We said this prayer after each group session with the patients who were struggling with addictions. The prayer reads, "Lord, grant me the serenity to accept the things I cannot change, the courage to change the things I can, and the wisdom to know the difference."

During your retreat allow yourself to be open to receiving whatever the Spirit has to offer you. Sit in silence and wait on your gift. I always invoke a prayer before and after my retreats; usually it is the Serenity Prayer. It holds me emotionally through my chaos; it grants me the serenity to remember that I indeed signed a sacred contract with my soul in attendance.

Below are a couple of my favorite quotes. These are lights of inspiration for me, and hopefully they will light your fire of desire for conscious living so you, too, can be purpose driven. Be sure to look at the end of the book for many more helpful resource suggestions.

If I had a magic wand, I'm not sure how often I would use it to help others because it is through our chaos, struggles, and challenges that we develop our true character. Going through the fire gives us a chance to practice Don Ruiz's four agreements from his book, *The Four Agreements: A Practical Guide to Personal Freedom:*[57]

1. Be impeccable with your word.
2. Don't take anything personally.
3. Don't make assumptions.
4. Always do your best.

My favorite quote when I get caught up in my self-made chaos is this:

ATTITUDE

I believe the single most significant decision I can make on a day-to-day basis is my choice of attitude.

It is more important than my past, my education, my bank roll, my successes or failures, fame or pain, what other people think of me or say about me my circumstances, or my position.

Attitude keeps me going or cripples my progress. It alone fuels my fire or assaults my hope.

When my attitudes are right there is no barrier too high, no valley too deep, no dream too extreme, no challenge too great for me.

—Charles Swindoll.[58]

I have a renewed attitude about life. I know that life is filled with choices all day, every day and it is our option to determine which choice will benefit or hinder our day. It is our choice to stay stuck in our woundology or become aware of our wombology and move beyond what is holding us back and soar into our future.

Epilogue

There are two essential breaths that each one of us will experience from the womb to the tomb.

1. We inhale to start life.
2. We exhale to end life.

In between those two essential breaths is what we call a life span or living. If I can help you breathe deeper and slower while living a zestful life between the inhale and exhale, I am living my purpose. If I can teach you to live the Serenity Prayer, I am on purpose. And if I can touch the hole in your heart and help you transform it into a whole heart, again I am on purpose. Thank you.

I am a passionate field hand for the universe, which means I am willing to do what I can, when I can, and where I can to help you find spiritual growth, emotional freedom, and mental clarity, which allows you to live a purpose-filled life. When this happens, your seven generations and my seven can become healing channels for others.

Life is not without challenges, struggles, and detours. Your attitude directs your aptitude and will help or hinder your choices. I chose to let my light shine, not blind, to live a golden life filled with opportunities, and to smile during my final exhale.

To your inhalations and exhalations,

Dr. C J

Too blessed to be depressed

About the Author

C J Johnson, PsyD, is a clinical psychologist, emotional freedom expert, life coach, and spiritual midwife. Throughout her more than fourteen years as an Adlerian therapist, she has encouraged others to follow their passion and fulfill their purpose. She lives in Georgia with her husband and is the mother of an adult son and daughter.

Contact:

C J Johnson, PsyD
You-Nique Wellness Psychotherapy
Stockbridge, GA 30281
E-mail: doctorcj@bellsouth.net

Appendix

My reframing of my father's detachment

WAVING IT OFF

I see Daddy dressed in his striped overalls wearing his baseball cap cocked arrogantly upward, carrying fishing poles with large hooks and red and white bobbins dobbing, minnows that swam in their own hole-filled bucket, and a pack of Lucky Strike cigarettes peering from his left pocket. Scents of Doublemint chewing gum, fish bait, and his Lucky Strikes all intermingled and announced it is time to go fishing. Yeah, that is one of my favorite images of my father.

The man I have to praise for teaching me detachment—how to be somewhere and not get too involved in what is going on for my self-preservation.

I praise him for teaching me how life is not fair. Some children have *Father Knows Best* for a daddy; others do not.

I praise him for teaching me how to handle not getting what I want when I want it—a bright, shiny red bicycle, for instance, because he does not want to spoil me.

I praise him for showing me how wonderful and committed my mom is. She is always there, listening and sacrificing for other's sake.

I praise him for teaching me how to set boundaries. Whenever I asked to do something with him, the answer was no.

I praise him for teaching me how to handle ridicule at an early age. Kids teased me about my father's "other" family.

I praise him for teaching me how to not take it personally. When he did more for them than for me, it was not about me.

I praise him for teaching me that others' mistakes are not my fault. It was his choice to turn right when he should have turned left.

I praise him for teaching me how to persevere. "Daddy, can I go? "No." Maybe next time he will say yes, so I just kept asking.

I praise him for helping me choose the perfect husband for me. He is so different from him.

Endnotes

Chapter 1: Womb-time Can Dictate a Lifetime

[1]   Chamberlain, *The Fetal Senses: A Classical View,* 18.

[2]   Verny, *The Secret Life of the Unborn Child,* 19.

[3]   Pearsall, *The Heart's Code: Tapping the Wisdom and Power of Our Heart Energy,* 19.

[4]   International Society of Prenatal and Perinatal Psychology and Medicine, *International Congress on The Anthropology and Psychology of Pregnancy and Birth,* 19.

[5]   Reiter, *Foetal Programming,* 19.

[6]   Upchurch, *Convicted in the Womb: One Man's Journey from Prisoner to Peacemaker,* 20.

[7]   King James Version, *The Holy Bible,* 20.

[8]   Northrup, *Mother-Daughter Wisdom: Creating a Legacy of Physical and Emotional Health,* 20.

[9]   Verny, *The Secret Life of the Unborn Child,* 22.

[10]   Kisilevsky et al., *"Effects of experience on fetal voice recognition,"* 22.

[11]   DeCasper, *Fetal Reactions to Recurrent Maternal Speech,* Infant Behavioral and Development, 22.

[12]   Wesson, *Brain Basics for the Teaching Professional,* 23.

[13]   Sontag, *Fels Longitudinal Study,* 23.

[14]   National Geographic Channel, *In the Womb.* London, 23.

Chapter 2: The Shaping of the Unborn

[15]   Myss, *Anatomy of the Spirit: The Seven Stages of Power and Healing,* 24.

16   Verny, *The Secret Life of the Unborn Child*, 25.

17   Ibid. *The Secret Life of the Unborn Child*, 25.

18   Bradshaw, *Healing the Shame That Binds You*, 28.

19   Glaser, *Monkey Do, Monkey See*, 28.

20   Bradshaw, *Healing the Shame that Binds You*, 20.

21   Northrup, *Mother-Daughter Wisdom*, 32.

22   Doi, *The Anatomy of Dependence*, 32.

23   Bowlby, *A Secure Base: Parent-Child Attachment and Healthy Human Development*, 33.

24   Ainsworth, *Patterns of Attachment: A Psychological Study of the Strange Situation*, 33.

25   Verny, *The Secret Life of the Unborn Child*, 34.

Chapter 3: Angry All the Time

26   Gray, *Men Are from Mars, Women Are from Venus, 37.*

27   Maslow et al., *New Knowledge in Human Values*, 42.

28   Hurston, *Anger*, 42.

29   Dayton, *The Soul's Companion: Connecting with the Soul through Daily Meditations, 43.*

30   Myss, *The Anatomy of the Spirit*, 44.

Chapter 4: Mind over Matter: What's in the Mind Matters

31   Zimbardo et al., *Psychology Core Concepts, 46.*

32   Ibid. *Psychology Core Concepts, 46.*

33   Braheny, *Mind, Body, Spirit: Connecting with Your Creative Self, 47.*

Chapter 5: Healing Memories

34   Braheny, *Mind, Body, Spirit: Connecting with Your Creative Self, 48.*

35   Verny, *Secret Life of the Unborn*, 48.

36   Ronald Gross, *Socrates' Way: Seven Master Keys to Using Your Mind to the Utmost, 49.*

37   Northrup, *Mother-Daughter Wisdom*, 50.

38   Jung, *Memories, Dreams, Reflections, 50.*

39   Myss, *Anatomy of the Spirit*, 51.

40   Shapiro, *Your Body Speaks Your Mind: Understanding How Your Thoughts and Emotions Affect Your Health, 51.*

Chapter 6: Warning Inner Child at Play

[41]   Bradshaw, *Healing the Shame that Binds You*, 56.
[42]   Ibid. *Healing the Shame that Binds You*, 56.
[43]   Missildine, *Your Inner Child of the Past*, 56.
[44]   Jung, *Memories, Dreams, Reflections*, 56.
[45]   Ibid. *Memories, Dreams, Reflections*, 57.

Chapter 7: Growing Beyond the PAST

[46]   Adler, *What Life Could Mean to You*, 64.
[47]   Grosskopf, *Forgive Your Parents, Heal Yourself: How Understanding Your Painful Family Legacy Can Transform Your Life*, 64.
[48]   Myss, *Anatomy of the Spirit*, 65.
[49]   Exley, *Mother's Notebook: For Personal Notes, Mementos, Recipes, or Home Planning*, 66.
[50]   Dayton, *The Magic of Forgiveness: Emotional Freedom and Transformation at Midlife*, 66.
[51]   Luft, *Group Processes: An Introduction to Group Dynamics*, 67.
[52]   Barnes, *Healing Ancient Wounds: The Renegade's Wisdom*, 68.
[53]   Gach, *Acupressure for Emotional Healing: Self-Care Guide for Trauma, Stress, and Common Emotional Imbalances*, 68.
[54]   Craig, *Emotional Freedom Technique*, 68.
[55]   Campbell, *We must be willing*, 69.
[56]   Williamson, *A Return to Love: Reflections on the Principles of a Course in Miracles*, 77.
[57]   Ruiz, *The Four Agreements: A Practical Guide to Personal Freedom*, 78.
[58]   Charles Swindoll, *Attitude*, 79.

Suggested Resources

READING

Bradshaw, John. *Homecoming: Reclaiming & Championing Your Inner Child.*
New York: Bantam Books, 1990.

Hay, Louise. *You Can Heal Your Life.* Carlsbad, Calif.: Hay House Publishing,
1999.

Levine, Peter. *Healing Trauma: A Pioneering Program for Restoring the Wisdom
of Your Body.* Boulder, Colo.: Sounds True Inc., 2005.

Nilsson, Lennart. *Life.* New York: Harry N. Abrams, Inc., 2006.

Osherson, Samuel. *Finding Our Fathers: The Unfinished Business of Manhood.*
New York: The Free Press, 1986.

Ruiz, Don Miguel, and Ruiz, Don Jose *The Four Agreements: Practical Guide
to Personal Freedom.* San Rafael, Calif.: Amber-Allen Publishing, 1997.

MUSIC

Cooper, Simon. *Music of the Womb*, Vol. II. Oreade Music, 2000.

Gordon, David, and Gordon, Steve. *Sacred Earth Drums,* Sequoia Records,
2004.

Hay, Louise. *Morning & Evening Meditations,* Hay House.

McNamara, Stevin. *Caroline Myss' Chakra Meditation Music,* Sounds True,
2003.

Nature's Retreat. *New Horizons,* Direct Source Products, Inc., 1998.

Sounds True. *Seeds of Awakening,* 2006.

Thompson, Jeffrey. *Healing Mind System, Brainwave Massage, Brainwave Suite,* The Relaxation Company.

DVDs

National Geographic Channel, *In the Womb,* The Pioneer Film & TV Productions, 2005.

National Geographic Channel, *Multiples in the Womb,* The Pioneer Film & TV Prod. 2006.

Web Sites
www.amazon.com
www.centerpointe.com
www.drnorthrup.com
www.emofree.com
www.hayhouse.com
www.innerhealingjourney.org
www.johnbradshaw.com
www.luciac.com
www.myss.com
www.myofascialrelease.com
www.therelaxationcompany.com
www.tiandayton.com
www.trvernymd.com

BODYWORK RESOURCES

Therapy on the Rocks
676 N. Highway 89A
Sedona, AZ 86336
(928) 282-3002

Myofascial Release Treatment Centers and Seminars
222 W. Lancaster Ave., Suite 100
Paoli, PA 19301
(800) 327-2425

Emotional Freedom Technique
P.O. Box 269
Coulterville, CA 95311

Bibliography

Adler, Alfred. *What Life Could Mean to You*. Center City, Minn.: Hazelden, 1998.

Ainsworth, Mary, Blehar, Mary, Waters, Everett, and Wall, Sally. *Patterns of Attachment: A Psychological Study of the Strange Situation*. Hillsdale, N.J.: Lawrence Erlbaum, 1979.

Barnes, John. *Healing Ancient Wounds: The Renegade's Wisdom*. Paoli, Pa.: Pennsylvania Rehabilitation Services, Inc., 2000.

Bowen, Murray, and Kerr, Michael. *Family Evaluation: An Approach on Bowen Theory*. New York: W.W. Norton and Company, 1988.

Bowlby, John. *A Secure Base: Parent-Child Attachment and Healthy Human Development*. New York: Basic Books, 1990.

Bradshaw, John. *Healing the Shame That Binds You,* revised and expanded ed. Deerfield Beach, Fla.: Health Communications, Inc., 2005.

Braheny, Mary, and Halperin, Diane. *Mind, Body, Spirit: Connecting with Your Creative Self*. Deerfield Beach, Fla.: Health Communications, Inc., 1989.

Capacchione, Lucia. *Recovery of Your Inner Child*. New York: Fireside, 1991.

Dayton, Tian. *The Soul's Companion: Connecting with the Soul through Daily Meditations*. Deerfield, Fla.: Health Communications Inc., 1995.

_____. *The Magic of Forgiveness: Emotional Freedom and Transformation at Midlife*. Deerfield, Fla.: Health Communications, Inc., 2003.

De Bono, Edward. *de Bono's Thinking Course*. New York: Facts on File Publications, 1985.

Doi, Takeo. *The Anatomy of Dependence*. New York: Kodansha International, 2002.

Exley, Helen. *Mother's Notebook: For Personal Notes, Mementos, Recipes or Home Planning*. Mount Kisco, N.Y.: Exley Publications Ltd., 1993.

Gach, Michael, and Henning, Beth. *Acupressure for Emotional Healing*. New York: Bantam Books, 2004.

Gray, John. *Men Are from Mars, Women Are from Venus*. New York: HarperCollins, 1992.

Grosskopf, Barry. *Forgive Your Parents, Heal Yourself*. New York: The Free Press, 1999.

Grun, Bernard. *The Timetables of History*. New York: Simon & Schuster, 1982.

Jennings, Peter, and Brewster, Todd. *The Century for Young People*. New York: Doubleday, 1999.

Jung, Carl, G. *Memories, Dreams, Reflections*. New York: Pantheon Books, 1963.

King James Version. *The Holy Bible*. New York: Thomas Nelson Publishers, 1977.

Kisilevsky, Barbara, Hains, S., Lee, K. Xie, X., Huang, H., et al., May 2003. "Effects of experience on fetal voice recognition," *Psychological Science* 14: 220–224.

Kosslyn, Stephen, and Rosenberg, Robin. *Fundamentals of Psychology: The Brain, the Person, the World*, second ed. Boston: Allyn & Bacon, 2005.

Luft, John. *Group Processes: An Introduction to Group Dynamics*. Palo Alto: National Press. 1966.

Maslow, Abraham et al., *New Knowledge in Human Values*. Chicago: Henry Regnery Company, 1959.

Matsakis, Aphrodite. *I Can't Get Over It*. Oakland: New Harbinger Publications, Inc., 1996.

Missildine, W. Hugh. *Your Inner Child of the Past*. New York: Pocket Books, 1963.

Myss, Caroline. *Anatomy of the Spirit: The Seven Stages of Power and Healing*. New York: Three Rivers Press, 1996.

National Geographic Channel. *In the Womb*, 2005.

Northrup, Christiane. *Mother-Daughter Wisdom: Creating a Legacy of Physical and Emotional Health*. New York: Bantam Dell, 2005.

Ruiz, Don. *The Four Agreements: A Practical Guide to Personal Freedom*. San Rafael, Calif.: Amber-Allen Publishing, 1997.

Shapiro, Debbie. *Your Body Speaks Your Mind: Understand How Your Thoughts and Emotions Affect Your Health*. London: Piatkus Books Ltd., 2005.

Stolley, Richard, and Chiu, Tony. *Life: Century of Change: America in Pictures, 1900–2000*. New York: Little, Brown and Company, 2000.

Upchurch, Carl. *Convicted in the Womb: One Man's Journey from Prisoner to Peacemaker*. New York: Bantam Books, 1996.

Verny, Thomas, and Kelly, John. *The Secret Life of the Unborn Child*. New York: Delta Book, 1981.

Williamson, Marianne. *A Return to Love: Reflections on the Principles of a Course in Miracles*. New York: HarperCollins, 1996.

Zimbardo, Philip, Johnson, Robert, and Weber, Ann. *Psychology: Core Concepts*, fifth ed. Boston: Allyn & Bacon, 2006.